MICROCOMPUTERS AND THE PRIVATE PRACTITIONER

Microcomputers

and the Private

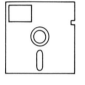

Practitioner

ROBERT M. PRESSMAN

DOW JONES-IRWIN
Homewood, Illinois 60430

© ROBERT M. PRESSMAN, 1984

All rights reserved. No part of this publication may be reproduced, stored in a retrieval system, or transmitted, in any form or by any means, electronic, mechanical, photocopying, recording, or otherwise, without the prior written permission of the copyright holder.

This publication is designed to provide accurate and authoritative information in regard to the subject matter covered. It is sold with the understanding that neither the author nor the publisher is engaged in rendering legal, accounting, or other professional service. If legal advice or other expert assistance is required, the services of a competent professional person should be sought.

From a Declaration of Principles jointly adopted by a Committee of the American Bar Association and a Committee of Publishers.

ISBN 0-87094-484-3

Library of Congress Catalog Card No. 83-73717

Printed in the United States of America

1 2 3 4 5 6 7 8 9 0 MP 1 0 9 8 7 6 5 4

DEDICATION

To Rose and Simon Pressman, my parents,
whose legacy of imagination and courage has been
the foundation of my journey through life.

SPECIAL RECOGNITION AND THANKS

To Ed Juge, for his visionary and trusting nature, without which this book might not have existed.

Preface

The world marveled at the mysterious machine called UNIVAC I. This electronic wonder, constructed in 1951, would fill the space of today's typical medical office. It consisted of hundreds of vacuum tubes and required a special environment that was maintained by several tons of air conditioning equipment. Scientific calculations that took hours, if not days, to do could now be made in seconds on this computer. That machine cost over $250,000. Now, some thirty years later, a $200 hand-held computer/calculator can do the same computations. The only difference is that the hand-held machine is faster and more reliable than its older sister.

The transition from vacuum tube to transistor to silicon chip has created a new technological age that most people have yet to comprehend. McLuhan has shown that faster forms of communication win out over more laborious forms, and this holds true for data storage/retrieval and computation. The question is not, "Will I ever use a microcomputer in my office?" but rather, "How soon will I be using a microcomputer in my office?" Advances in computer technology are occurring at a lightning-fast rate.

The practitioner who fails to understand the impact of computer technology may soon be surpassed by his more enlightened competitors. They will be using computers for data base diagnoses, lickety-split billing to patients and insurance companies, and word processing techniques that will be accomplished with far less effort and far greater efficiency than have previously been available. Even at present, the costs for systems with these capabilities are modest. Although it is possible to spend $30,000 for a combination of hardware and software, *complete* top-of-the-line systems can be purchased for under $12,500. Effective, but less complete, systems can be purchased for around $3,000 to $5,000.

Microcomputers and the Private Practitioner is designed both for the practitioner who has a fundamental knowledge of computer science and for the practitioner who has no background at all. Chapter 1 lets the uninititated know what to expect from an office computer. Chapters 2 and 3 discuss critical programs in detail. Chapter 4 describes a model private practice system. Chapter 5 gives hints on how to convert to a computer system. Chapter 6 tells how to avoid the worst kind of computer disaster. Chapter 7 destroys some old myths. Chapter 8 walks the reader through a typical day with an office computer. Chapter 9 suggests ways of preparing the reader and staff for the changes to be ushered in by the computer. Chapter 10 suggests how the reader may deal with consultants. Chapter 11 provides the practitioner with enough detail to set up a complete system herself. Chapter 12 demonstrates an alternative to on-site computer use. Chapter 13 reveals the "secrets" of data base management. Chapter 14 demonstrates methods by which the computer can be used to increase the practitioner's income. And finally, Chapter 15 looks at multi-user systems and the future.

Microcomputers and the Private Practitioner is for practitioners in the broad spectrum of the allied health fields. This includes physicians, dentists, and mental health practitioners. Computer developments are continuous in all of these fields and are indicative both of the current demand of the market and of what the demand is expected to be. If you are contemplating the purchase of a computer system for your practice or want an understanding of how your system may be utilized more effectively to build your practice, read on.

ACKNOWLEDGMENTS

Microcomputers and the Private Practitioner was special for me in that it required the inclusion of more technical information than did previous works. In its development I sought technical assistance from many computer-related companies. A few companies rose to the occasion to an extraordinary degree. I would like to acknowledge them here, as their help was invaluable. Although most of the "giants" seemed too busy or preoccupied, the response from Radio Shack exceeded my wildest expectations. At the national level, Ed Juge, director, computer merchandising, provided continual information about updates in the field and opportunities for hands-on experience with Radio Shack hardware and software developments. Janet Brauhn, executive secretary, from the "15th Floor" of One Tandy Center, Fort Worth, helped facilitate and coordinate Radio Shack's efforts to assist me.

At the local level, Tom King, the manager of the computer department, was always available to answer questions and to provide technical assistance and advice at our office. Tobey Richards and Tony Volpe, of the East Providence and Providence computer centers, provided my staff and me with about 100 hours of instruction.

Much appreciation to my publisher, Dow Jones-Irwin, for providing me with the password to access its sister company, Dow Jones News Retrieval Service (with the instructions "Don't use it too much"). Thanks also to Theo Jolosky of Interpretive Scoring Systems of NCS for introducing me to Arion, National Computer System's psychological telecomputing system.

Three other individuals have been helpful to me in each of the private practice management books that I have written. Deborah Brennan, then a reference librarian and now the head librarian of the North Kingstown Free Library, turned a small library, located in the Rhode Island fishing port of Wickford, into an international depot for interlibrary loans. I doubt whether I could have gotten better service if I lived next to the Library of Congress.

Tim Jackson and Safeguard Business Systems have been a generous source of information regarding developments in the field of business management. They have shown a constant willingness to share information and to test out new concepts as they have been developed in my books.

Susan Whitney, my trusty secretary over the years has been a pivotal person in the production of these books. She helped bang out the earlier books with a Selectric typewriter, and with this one she became an adept computer manager and word processing operator.

And finally, I would like to acknowledge the support and assistance of my wife, Stephanie Pressman, an author in her own right. Her advice regarding style was invaluable, as were her words of encouragement as the book progressed.

The reader may note that there is considerable but not exclusive use of the feminine pronoun throughout the book. I felt (or hoped) that the nonconventional use of the gender pronoun would: (1) raise the level of consciousness regarding the professional role of women, (2) not hurt sales of the book.

There is a brain twister that goes as follows:

> A five-year-old child is rushed to the emergency room. Although the ER doctor is not the boy's father, it is the hospital's policy that doctors

cannot operate on immediate members of their family. Therefore, the doctor is forbidden to intervene with the boy. What is the relationship between the physician and the child? The answer is printed below.

If you got the answer right (which I didn't) then you will probably sail through the book without batting an eye at the mixture of pronouns.

ʇǝɥʇoɯ s,ʎoq ǝɥʇ sı ɹoʇɔop ǝɥ⊥

Robert M. Pressman

Contents

1. What to Expect from a Computer   **1**
What Do Computers Do Well? *Billing. Typewriting. Scoring. Tracking Accounts.* Should You Own a Computer? *Two Ways to Go.*

2. The Most Important Program   **5**
The Fundamental Software Package. MOS Files: *Practice File. Patient File. Diagnostic File. Procedure File. Transaction File.* Report Formats: *Financial Reports. Demographic Reports.* Sorting. Label Printing. Other Considerations: *One or Two Disks. Doomsday Programs.* Implementing the System.

3. The "Other" Programs   **17**
Software. Medical Office System. Word Processing. Additional Word Processing Software. General Ledger. Data Base Management. Accounts Payable and Payroll Systems. Communication Software. Electronic Spread Sheets. Accounts Receivable.

4. The System   **27**
The System. Keyboard: *Configuration. Feel. Detachability.* CPU. Memory and Storage: *Disk Drives. How Much Storage Do You Need?* Printer. Printers for the Medical Office. Video Display: *Radiation.* Communication Hardware. Other Items: *Blank Diskettes. Storage Boxes. Cables. Maintenance and Cleaning Supplies. Antistatic Supplies and Equipment. Dustcovers. Power Line Protectors. Printer Tractor. Printer Table. Computer Table. Fanfold Folders. Data Racks. Print Ruler. Labels and Felt Tip Pens. Data Trays.*

5. Starting Up the MOS   **47**
Take 90 Days. When's the Best Time to Start? Time Reallocation: *Training. Practice. Routine Use.* The Agony of Defeat and the Ecstasy of Victory: *Previous Accounts. Quirks in Recording and Amending Transactions. Learning Systems Commands and Techniques. Reporting Techniques. Aging and Dunning Messages.* Insurance Forms. Adequate Supplies.

6. Backups   55
A Short Story with a Long Legacy. How to Make Efficient Backups: *Floppy Disk Backups. Hard Disk Backups. Long-Range Backups.*

7. Myths   59
The Purchase of a Computer System Follows a Scientific Study. It's Expensive. It's Inexpensive. It's Complicated. It's Simple. It Saves Time. Hard Disk Drive Will Make Your Computer as Fast as a Mainframe. Turnkey Operations Are Trouble-Free.

8. A Typical Day with the Computer   65
A Typical Day. Interview with Ms. Hennessy, Computer User. Interview with Dr. Reed, Computer Owner.

9. Preparing Self and Staff   79
Preparation: *Should You Learn How to Program? Minimize Changes.* Prior Involvement of Staff: *Discussion. What Training Is Needed?* Sequence of Ordering: *Insurance Forms. Invoice Forms. Other Supplies.* Physical Considerations: *Electrical Demands. Furniture Configuration. Lighting.* Hang Loose.

10. Turnkey Systems   85
A Matter of Finances. Guidelines: *Custom-Made. Support. Costs. Time. Proximity. Financial Stability. Labeling Oranges and Apples.*

11. Your Own Turnkey Operation for under $12,500   91
Do It Yourself: *Radio Shack. The Catalog. Seven Fundamental Requirements. Close to Home.* Instruction: *Operator's Course. Word Processing Course. Data Base Course.* Equipment: *Computer. Keyboard. Floppy Disk Drives. Operating System. Hard Disk Drive. Printer. Bidirectional Tractors. Modem. Furniture.* Software: *Medical Office System. Scripsit. Scripsit Spelling and Hyphenation Dictionary. Profile Plus. Visi-Calc.* Supplies. Avoiding Downtime: *Service. Service Contracts. Maintenance. Support. When Things Go Haywire.* The Shopping List.

12. Alternatives to the Computer   109
Alternatives. Advantages: *Investment. Broader Programs. Freedom from Troubleshooting. Cost Containment. Staff Training.* Disadvantages: *Lack of Spontaneity. Program Modification and Development. Insurance Statements. Word Processing.*

13. **Helping the Computer Make Money for You** — 117
    The Computer Can Make Money for You. Optimal Use. Stimulating Patient/Client Interest: *Recall. Follow-Up. Letters to Referral Sources. Mailings to Potential Referral Sources.* Billing and Collection: *Billing Dates and Procedures. Tracking Accounts.* Ancillary Use of the Computer.

14. **My Name Is Fink** — 129
    My Name Is Fink. How Does It Work? Data Bases: *Who's Who in the Zoo. Recreational Data Base.* Readable Data Bases: *Serious Data Bases.* Time and Charges. Efficiency. The Future.

15. **Multi-User Systems** — 135
    Picture This. Ramifications. Advantages: *Speed. Multiple Access. Automatic Functions. Software Savings. Hardware Savings.* Disadvantages: *Cost. Speed. Confidentiality.* The Future.

GLOSSARY — 141

REFERENCES — 147

ANNOTATED BIBLIOGRAPHY — 149

APPENDIX A: Examples of Computer Reports on Practice Activity — 155

APPENDIX B: Health Insurance Claim Form—HCFA 1500/CHAMPUS 501 (C–3) — 163

APPENDIX C: Practice Analysis Utilizing Computer Graphics — 165

APPENDIX D: Example of Computer Scored and Interpreted MMPI — 169

APPENDIX E: Sample Report of Millon Behavior Health Inventory — 179

INDEX — 187

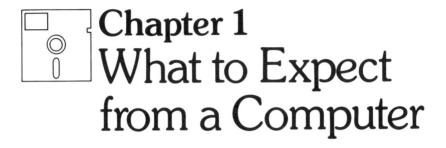
Chapter 1
What to Expect from a Computer

WHAT DO COMPUTERS DO WELL?
   Billing
   Typewriting
   Scoring
   Tracking Accounts
SHOULD YOU OWN A COMPUTER?
   Two Ways to Go

WHAT DO COMPUTERS DO WELL?

What can you expect from a computer? What are the practical applications for the private practitioner? To derive an answer, one only has to ask what computers do well: *they perform tedious and repetitive tasks with lightning speed and high accuracy.* They therefore have considerable application in the business management of a private practice. The following tedious and repetitive tasks are performed in such a practice: (1) billing patients and third-party payers; (2) typewriting letters, reports and envelopes; (3) scoring test protocols; and (4) tracking accounts receivable and accounts payable. Let's look at each task briefly.

Billing

Billing is a largely repetitive procedure. The information for billing is stored and re-stored many times. The first place it may appear is on a patient intake sheet. It is then transferred to a ledger card and to "day sheets," possibly photocopied on a billing sheet, most certainly written or typed on a third-party payment insurance form. Other data regarding diagnosis and services rendered may also be entered a number of times. On the computer, information is entered only once. Afterward, it will automatically appear on the ledger card, data sheet, insurance forms, transaction slips, or whatever other ancillary programs permit the transfer of data. Whether information is entered into a computer or onto a handwritten data sheet, initial entry takes the same time. However, once the information has been entered, the picture changes dramatically. Consider that most computer programs produce 50 fully typed insurance forms, everything in the right place, in less than 30 minutes; the operator activates the program with perhaps three or four keystrokes and then goes on to do something else. Using a typewriter, most secretaries would require more than eight hours to complete 50 insurance forms.

Typewriting

The jargon for this term is word processing. Few letters or reports go out on the first draft. Hence, most letter and report writing is a repetitive procedure. If a corrected copy of the first draft comes back, this means either retyping the original draft or making erasures on it and making do with however it can be doctored up. Even after the best of efforts in proofreading, the revised letter or report may go out with errors that have eluded the secretary and the practitioner. In computer typewriting, however, a draft first appears on a video screen. Words may be changed and manipulated instantly. Since whatever mistakes made can easily be corrected, the secretary feels free to type rapidly. Various proofreading programs are available that will quickly appraise spelling and grammar. When this has been done, the draft may be "typed" or printed at an average rate of one page per 40 seconds. Such drafts are usually produced on inexpensive computer paper, sometimes in long runs of multiple letters to be read over by the practitioner, given back to the secretary, and run off as final drafts at a rate of one to two pages per minute. Envelopes may be printed by referring to electronic files of names and addresses.

Scoring

In the last year or two there has been an increase in the development of software to assist the practitioner in administering and scoring psychological test protocols. Here, whether the practitioner is using the Wechsler Scales, Rorschach, or the MMPI, conclusions are based on numerical calculations. The computer not only makes the calculations but has even been used in the actual administration of the tests.

Tracking Accounts

Keeping an accounts receivable ledger and dunning system is another task that the computer does well. Gone are the days of having to look at ledger cards one at a time to determine how old each balance is and whether or not the age and amount of the balance are sufficient for some type of dunning action. Once the criteria for taking various types of actions have been set, patients may be classified in accordance with these criteria. Falling into one classification may entail the placement of a sticker saying "past due" on the patient's bill. Falling into another classification may entail the mailing of a personal letter to the patient discussing the age and balance of the account. These are tasks that the computer does with great facility. It is able to generate detailed accounts receivable reports of several hundred patients within minutes. Combined with word processing formats, it can generate both dunning notices and "personalized" letters. For example, in less than 40 minutes the computer can generate individually typed personal letters to a hundred patients, giving each of them specific information about their accounts.

The practitioner who is so inclined may apply similar efficiency to keeping track and control of accounts payable and tying this format into a check-writing procedure.

Anyone who keeps a check register or books knows well the tedium and repetition involved. There are problems in having computers do the actual writing of checks, but the process of tracking assets, liabilities, receivables, and payables is one that invariably involves storing the same information in multiple formats, performing calculations on it, and producing reports from it.

The computer has the advantage of being able to take the data entered only once and to distribute it and calculate it to produce checks, check registers, balance sheets, billings, and prompts to payables—all with a speed that defies imagination.

SHOULD YOU OWN A COMPUTER?

The question, then, is whether you should get a computer and, if so, what kind should you get and what is the best way to get it?

Two Ways to Go

One way to go is with a turnkey operation, and the other is to acquire and implement the system yourself. In a turnkey operation a consultant company works with you to determine your needs and to provide equipment, software, training, and support. In other words, you pay the money and then all you have to do is turn the key to get going. There is a premium of about 50 percent for this type of service. For many practitioners, it is well worth an additional $5,000 or $10,000 to have a system operational and debugged. But for many others, there is a real incentive in creating and implementing a system that is unique and quasi do-it-yourself.

The following chapters are designed to help the practitioner decide whether or not to get a computer. But they also provide information regarding the types of programs and equipment needed, how they are utilized in a practice, and what costs are involved. Read on!

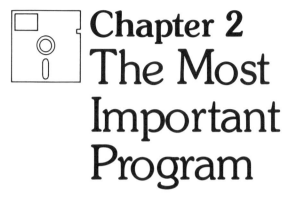

Chapter 2
The Most Important Program

THE FUNDAMENTAL SOFTWARE PACKAGE
MOS FILES
    Practice File
    Patient File
    Diagnostic File
    Procedure File
    Transaction File
        Charge Transactions
        Payment Transactions
REPORT FORMATS
    Financial Reports
        Insurance Forms
        Patient Statements
        Financial Recaps
    Demographic Reports
SORTING
LABEL PRINTING
OTHER CONSIDERATIONS
    One or Two Disks
    Doomsday Programs
IMPLEMENTING THE SYSTEM

THE FUNDAMENTAL SOFTWARE PACKAGE

The fundamental software package in a doctor's office is usually referred to as an MOS (medical office system). A dental office system could be referred to as a DOS and a psychological office system as a POS, but since there are very few differences in the major parts of these systems, for simplicity every office system discussed in this book will be referred to as an MOS.

Whether you choose to do it yourself or purchase a turnkey operation, your MOS should perform the basic and integrated financial functions explained below. There are additional functions that an MOS might perform (for example, word processing), but these are icing on the cake and are not absolutely necessary. They will be discussed elsewhere. In this chapter the *principal* MOS components will be explored. By the time you finish reading it, you should have a good sense of the type of MOS software you will need for your practice.

Most practitioners have enough computer savvy to know that when you "talk" to a computer you must be *very* specific. Seemingly simple tasks are often quite complex. Billing, for example, may seem to have only a few variables. In fact, several dozen steps involving various segments of information must often be taken before bills can be sent out. These segments will involve information stored in the manner described below.

MOS FILES

All MOS packages comprise five types of information or "files": the practice file, the patient file, the procedure file, the diagnostic file and the transaction file. Depending on how the program is written, these five files may be made to interact to store and produce a variety of reports. In computerese, a bill or invoice is one type of "report" format.

Practice File

The practice file usually consists of the following segments: the name and address of the practice; the names of the participating doctors and their identifying numbers such as the social security number or the federal employer number; and how billing and dunning should be handled (e.g., billing frequency and dunning messages to be placed automatically on designated invoices after 30-, 60-, 90-, or 120-day periods).

Patient File

The patient file contains the following segments: the patient's name, home address, occupation, work address, and telephone numbers. It also includes information necessary for filing insurance claims, such as the name of the insurance company, the owner of the policy, and the relevant contract and group numbers. Billing codes are recorded: Who is responsible for payment—the insurance company, the patient, two insurance companies? Should dunning information be automatically printed on the patient statements? Should a statement be withheld from printing for some reason? Should the account be placed in collection status? Most of these questions are answered by simple one-letter keystrokes, and the answers are stored in the patient's record until the information is updated. What other types of information may be recorded on the patient's record depends on the nature of the software program. Many programs permit the recording of medications and the dates they were prescribed so as to ensure automatic patient recall if necessary.

A patient record will be made interactive with several files. For example, a patient's record may contain information from the transaction file, such as outstanding balances due from the insurance company or the patient.

Diagnostic File

The diagnostic file may be a user-created list of diagnoses used in the practice. Some programs have prelisted diagnostic categories and codes. However, as diagnostic categories and codes are often updated, it is best to have a diagnostic file that can be altered by the user. Typically, there are four or five segments to this list. The first is a user number assigned to a particular diagnosis. If you use 30 diagnostic categories in your practice, the first one you list would have the "code" number 1, no matter what the ICDA or DMS III code may be. The number is for your quick reference. The second segment is a description of the diagnosis, such as anxiety neurosis. The third, fourth, or even fifth segments are the codes assigned for these diagnoses by ICDA, DSM III, and/or Medicare. Again, this file may become interactive with other files, including the patient record.

Procedure File

In this file, as in the diagnostic file, the doctor may assign her own numbers to frequently used procedures. The procedures may be described (for example, "Amalgam restoration—one surface" or "Psychotherapy—50 minutes"). Code numbers for procedures that conform to ICDA or Medicare standards are also used. This file may also record the usual charge for each procedure. Once the number of the procedure is entered on the patient's record, correct procedure codes and charges are automatically printed on the patient's bill or insurance form. Of course, a good program would permit the practitioner to override the standard charges when indicated.

Transaction File

This is probably the most important aspect of the MOS and the one most likely to result in user disappointment. Although transactions have many nuances, essentially there are only two types: charges and payments. From a bookkeeping point of view, a charge and a payment are two separate transactions even though they may be stored on the same line.

Charge Transactions. There are eight elements to a charge: date of service, place of service, doctor performing service, diagnosis, procedure, number of times procedure was performed, charge for procedure, and responsibility for payment (insurance company or patient). The diagnosis is sometimes stored on the charge record because third-party payers often demand that procedures be related to diagnosis.

Payment Transactions. Records of payment transactions contain the following information: date of payment, the payer (insurance company or patient), and amount of payment. Payment transactions may have other necessary nuances. How these are handled will depend largely on the program. They consist of the following: (1) modifications that may be made at the time of entry, particularly on the charge file (for example a charge for a standard procedure may be altered); (2) notes that may have to be added to the invoice for the benefit of the patient or the insurance company (such notes are typically entered in the transaction file); (3) adjustments or write-offs that may be necessary (adjustments are usually made when errors have occurred on the charge side of the transaction file); and (4) an audit trail of any adjustment that is left to prevent tampering (the date of service and the charge may be adjusted, but to prevent tampering the invoice line cannot be erased).

A separate aspect of the MOS involves the manner in which the information stored in the files is reported.

REPORT FORMATS

The term *report format* refers to any method by which the computer tabulates, collates, and presents information from various files. The printing of insurance forms (one of the most critical report features of the MOS) consists of taking information from all the files—practice, patient, diagnostic, procedure, and transaction files—and arranging the data so that they fall in the correct spaces of the insurance form. The printing of mailing labels, a convenient feature of some MOS packages, is also a kind of report format. In this case, limited information from the patient file is formatted so that it will print on labels inserted in the printer. Apart from their use in producing various billing forms—invoices, patient statements, insurance forms—report formats may be used to present a myriad of information.

The following vignette comes from a dentist who recently converted to computer usage. It gives some idea of the reporting power of the MOS.

> When I ordered my first box of green bar [refers to computer paper with faint horizontal green bars to make reading of numerical information easier], I thought I would splurge and get the "big carton" of 3,500 pages. Upon placing the order, I was asked quite sincerely, "Will that be enough?" Little did I know then of the computer's ability to calculate and print aspects of my practice from every angle and with detail beyond imagination. Next time I'm asked if that will be enough, my answer will be, "Yes, for this week."

Although the account is somewhat exaggerated, it contains more than a kernel of truth. Some of the report features of MOS packages are listed below. MOS reports may be automatically tied to certain features (for example, ledger posting invariably produces details regarding the transactions posted). Depending on the demands and curiosity of the operator, reports may be modified to include less or more detail. Report forms generally fall within two categories: financial and demographic.

Financial Reports

Insurance Forms. One of the most important features of an MOS is insurance form reporting. A big plus is having a program that the user may easily modify to accommodate different types of insurance forms. A psychotherapist from New England aptly describes the need for a user-modifiable MOS.

> I cannot imagine using an MOS that does not have a variable insurance form feature. In the state where I practice, the universal insurance form required by Blue Cross/Blue Shield is company supplied. Although one set of forms may look identical to another, all one has to do is have the horror of printing a complete batch of forms to find that the information appears to be coming out on the wrong place.
>
> Not long ago, Blue Cross/Blue Shield sent me a carton of 1,000 forms of HCFA 1500/CHAMPUS 501 (C-2) rather than HCFA 1500/CHAMPUS 501 (C-3). Because my MOS can be modified, I was able to produce the new forms in relatively short order. The alternative would have been days of scurrying around (that's if I were lucky) to acquire the forms compatible with my existing program and then to be subjected to the possibility that the insurance company would reject my efforts because the other form would not be "acceptable."
>
> In my practice I use three formats. One, a universal form where there is no disability involved; two, a universal form where there is disability involved, requiring the inclusion of special information; and three, a universal form for CHAMPUS. CHAMPUS seems to come up with a new regulation at least every six months for what kind of data it wants where. If you do a large volume with CHAMPUS, I would advise against acquiring an MOS package that does not provide for easy reforming of insurance forms!

Patient Statements. The need for user modification of the patient statement is usually not great. Software companies have designed statement programs to print on standard forms (see Figure 2-1). If worst comes to worst, one could always have a

FIGURE 2–1
Statement*

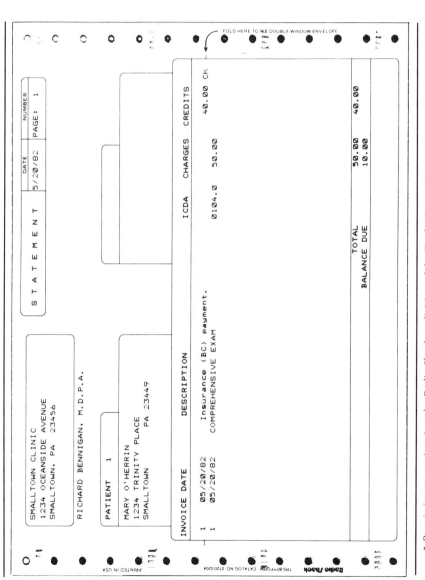

*Permission to reprint given by Radio Shack, a division of the Tandy Corporation.

form printed to conform to the computer program, rather than vice versa. In modifiable programs the practitioner may choose to suppress diagnostic descriptions and codes normally required by insurance companies. This information is sometimes confusing to the patient. Because diagnostic codes are numerical which may have two decimal places, the patient may confuse them with charges.

It is a convenience to have statements aged and to be able to print dunning messages related to the age of the statements. The dunning messages are usually stored in the practice file and merged automatically with the statement program. Typical messages might be as follows:

30 days: Past due.
60 days: Past due, second notice.
90 days: Account seriously past due. Payment today would be appreciated.
120 days: Final notice on past-due account.

Some programs also permit a universal and changeable message to be printed at each statement time. The message might be a season's greeting or a general statement about fee changes.

Financial Recaps. Reports may be developed on a wide front of financial variables, including the aging of accounts, the status of charges and payments and write-offs or other adjustments on a per patient, per day, per month, or per year basis. Such reports may be given in the form of figures or graphs.

Demographic Reports

Patient and general practice information may be extracted and given in report form. Typical reports might consist of telephone and address listings of each patient and an accounting of each diagnosis and procedure used. See Figure 2–2 and Figure 2–3.

SORTING

Most MOS programs permit the sorting of records by user-defined variables. A typical sort might be all patients with a balance of

FIGURE 2-2
Procedure File Report

Thu May 20 1982

SELECTED: ALL

MEDICAL OFFICE SYSTEM
PROCEDURE FILE REPORT

Page 1

C P T Code Modifier	Medicare Code	Procedure Number	Standard Charge	DESCRIPTION	Type of Service	Month to Date Times	Month to Date Amount	Year to Date Times	Year to Date Amount
90001		00001	50.00	COMPREHENSIVE EXAM	1	3	150.00	3	150.00
88150	90	00002	11.00	PAP SMEAR	5	1	11.00	1	11.00
90070		00003	22.00	OFFICE VISIT	1	2	44.00	2	44.00
90000		00004	35.00	GYNECOLOGICAL EXAM	1	2	70.00	2	70.00
59411		00005	675.00	OBSTETRICAL CARE, ROUTINE	1				
		00006		OFFICE VISIT FOR OB CARE	1				
59501		00007	900.00	OBSTETRICAL CARE, C-SECTION	1				
59000		00008	35.00	AMNIOCENTESIS	1				
90040		00010	30.00	PRENATAL/POSTPARTUM VISIT	1				
76805 26		00011	25.00	SONOGRAPHY	4				
88310	90	00012	15.00	TISSUE STUDY	5	1	25.00	1	25.00
85015		00013	12.00	CBC	0	1	15.00	1	15.00
81005		00014	12.00	CBC - WITHOUT DIFFERENTIAL	5				
81000		00015	18.00	UA, ROUTINE	5	1	18.00	1	18.00
85050		00016	12.00	UA, COMPLETE	0				
85055		00017	15.00	HEMOGLOBIN	0				
83168		00018	20.00	HEMATOCRIT	0				
85590		00019	15.00	PREGNANCY TEST	5				
86007		00021	18.00	PLATELET COUNT	0				
85660		00022	25.00	SICKLE CELL PREP	5				
86410		00023	25.00	SEROLOGY (RPR)	5				
86418		00024	20.00	SEROLOGY (RPR), PREMARITAL	5	1	20.00	1	20.00
84330	90	00025	50.00	GLUCOSE, FBS, or FBS-2 hr.	5				
84345	90	00026	65.00	GLUCOSE TOLERANCE - 3 hr.	5				
80329		00027		GLUCOSE TOLERANCE - 4,5,6 hr.	5				
		00028		CONSULTATION DURING SURGERY	3				
71022 26		00029	40.00	X-RAY CHEST-OPLIQUE PROJECT'N	4				
83400	90	00030		THYROID PROFILE- T3,T4,T7,PBI	5				
				BALANCE FORWARD					
						12	353.00	12	353.00

Permission to reprint given by Radio Shack, a division of the Tandy Corporation.

FIGURE 2-3
Patient File Report

```
                        M E D I C A L   O F F I C E   S Y S T E M
                                     PATIENT FILE REPORT

Thu May 20 1982                                                                          Page   1

SELECTED:  ALL

PATIENT    PATIENT'S NAME     ADDRESS             CITY        STATE   ZIP    HOME PHONE      WORK PHONE
NUMBER                                                                CODE
------    --------------     -------             ----        -----   ----   ----------     ----------
00001     MARY    O'HERRIN   1234 TRINITY PLACE  SMALLTOWN    PA      23449  555-232-7777    555-233-8681
00002     HOLLY   DOTSON     9385 RUTLAND        SMALLTOWN    PA      23455  321-567-8901
00003     GLADYS  SPARKS     3624 BORDEAUX       SMALLTOWN    PA      23455  321-443-4398    321-447-1784 X11
00004     ALICE   HOUSEMAN   22 BROOKSIDE        SMALLTOWN    PA      23454  321-655-432E    321-432-9871
00005     MELINDA OMENS      6781 PECAN          SMALLTOWN    PA      23444  321-123-1231
00006     BEATRICE CONSTANTINO 5228 GREENLEE     SMALLTOWN    PA      23456  321-377-2184    321-488-2916
00007     WANDA   KYBER      8988 CORNERSTONE    SMALLTOWN    PA      23459  321-289-1984    321-483-2111
00008     ROBIN   WHITBECK   7388 SALEM AVENUE   SMALLTOWN    PA      23455  321-654-7171    321-773-1994
00009     JAMIE   ANTHONY    2345 OVERHILL LANE  SMALLTOWN    PA      23449  321-533-9216
00010     GISELLE GASPAR     2711 PLANTATION     SMALLTOWN    PA      23358  321-993-5454    321-488-8952
```

Permission to reprint given by Radio Shack, a division of the Tandy Corporation.

over $100 for more than 60 days. Once defined, the sorts may be viewed on the screen as individual records, printed in one of the above report formats, or merged with a word processing program to produce letters to the individuals sorted. Other helpful sort variables might include zip code, medication, diagnosis, procedure, date last seen, and referral source.

LABEL PRINTING

This is a minor but helpful program. It facilitates mailings to selected patients. Patient variables are defined (e.g., any patient with a balance), and labels are produced for those patients to be used later in conjunction with a form letter.

OTHER CONSIDERATIONS

One or Two Disks

If you'll be working in floppy and have a small to medium-sized practice, then it is an advantage to house the MOS program on a single diskette. Some programs require housing on two diskettes. This is inconvenient, as backups must be made in pairs and an extra disk drive is needed to do word processing merges. With hard disk operations, this distinction is of no significance, as all application programs are permanently transferred to the hard disk drive.

Doomsday Programs

If the program fails to let you know when the data banks (files) are filled up, new material is recorded over old material, resulting in permanent data loss. It's hard to believe that any software manufacturer would let this happen, but stories still circulate about such occurrences.

IMPLEMENTING THE SYSTEM

There are five ways of implementing the MOS. The first is to have a good consulting firm develop a customized software package for you. This is expensive. The second is to put together a series of prepackaged programs yourself. This is inexpensive but hectic. The third is to purchase a turnkey operation, which tends to be expensive. The fourth is to create your own programs from scratch; this may leave you with little time to devote to your practice. And the fifth is to purchase an over-the-counter prepackaged MOS that can fulfill most of your MOS needs at relatively low cost. In addition, there are many ways in which an MOS can be implemented by using a combination of consultation and do-it-yourself.

The following chapters tell you: (1) what else you may need to acquire, (2) how to do it yourself, (3) how to have it done for you.

Chapter 3
The "Other" Programs

SOFTWARE
MEDICAL OFFICE SYSTEM
WORD PROCESSING
ADDITIONAL WORD PROCESSING
  SOFTWARE
GENERAL LEDGER
DATA BASE MANAGEMENT
ACCOUNTS PAYABLE AND PAYROLL
  SYSTEMS
COMMUNICATION SOFTWARE
ELECTRONIC SPREAD SHEETS
ACCOUNTS RECEIVABLE

SOFTWARE

There are several software categories that are essential for private practice management. The Medical Office System is often a hybrid of an accounts receivable program and a data base management program. In addition to this package, word processing and general ledger programs will be needed. Some MOS packages include these programs. Software categories that are very helpful, but not absolutely essential, for a basic operation are: financial spread sheet, communication packages, data base management systems, accounts payable, and payroll.

MEDICAL OFFICE SYSTEM

The Medical Office System (or psychological or dental office system) is the pivotal software package. Usually, it consists of hybrids of several packages or programs. It may even include some or all of the features in the other packages discussed below. As indicated in Chapter 2, it should be able to store, integrate, display, and/or print at least the following:

1. The practice file: Information about the practice (e.g., names of doctors, frequency of billing, and dunning messages).
2. The patient file: Demographic and insurance information relating to the patients.
3. The procedure file: Descriptions and codes of procedures commonly used in the practice.
4. The diagnostic file: Diagnostic categories, descriptions, and codes used in the practice.
5. The transaction file: Information regarding charges made to patients and payments made by patients or insurance companies.

The manner in which the MOS provides for ease of entry, correction, and reporting is as important as the categories themselves. Minimally, an MOS should be able to process the above information and print insurance forms and patient statements automatically after being instructed to do so with a few simple keystrokes. Detailed reporting about accounts receivable is another critical feature. Most systems will detail financial information about the charge and payment status of patients and groups of patients as well as the financial productivity of physicians. The inclusion of word processing and general ledger systems with the MOS or their inclusion in the MOS can be a convenience but is not essential.

WORD PROCESSING

Most practices have the need to produce reports and letters, though some practices produce many more than others. Practices that depend on referrals from primary care practitioners or perform insurance-related work tend to make greater use of word processing. By now, you know that *word processing* is a fancy term for the cycle of writing or dictating, typing, correcting, and retyping.

The primary function of word processing software is to facilitate text correction and manipulation, with the final step performed by a high-speed printer. If purchased when the computer is procured, the software and printer to produce letter quality adds a cost of $1,500 to a package that would otherwise include only a computer and a dot matrix printer. Any practice that generates 10 or more letters or reports a week will benefit from this add-on. It is difficult to justify the cost for practices that produce fewer than three letters or reports a week. For practices generating three to nine letters or reports a week, the decision to add on a letter-quality word processor will have more to do with aesthetics than economy. The unspoken advantage of a good word processing system (WPS) is that it assists the practitioner in producing *better* correspondence. Because a WPS permits text changes to be made quickly, there is less hesitancy about changing a word or two in order to improve a report. Without such a system, the doctor will often hesitate to make even minor changes because this might necessitate the tedious retyping of an entire page. Better-quality correspondence and reports reflect well on a practice. If top-notch correspondence is important to you and you produce three to nine letters or reports a week—add on a WPS.

It has been said that all owners of word processing software feel that their package is the best in the world. This devotion stems from a lack of opportunity to make comparisons and from the fact that nearly any word processor is far superior to any typewriter. Many word processing programs are available, and at some level one may be better than another. In the final analysis, problems in documentation and presentation will be overcome by the operator and the WPS will be learned with great facility. There are, however, basic functions that a WPS should perform, and since word processing programs are sold by the pound, so to speak, one should expect to pay about $400 retail for a thorough program.

The most fundamental WPS permits the entry of all keyboard letters and figures, upper- and lowercase, with a maximum column width of 80 characters and an automatic wraparound feature. This feature allows the operator to enter text without having to hit a return key at the end of each line. A partial word at the end of the line is automatically taken to start a new line. In addition, a WPS should be able to easily insert, delete, move, and copy characters, words, sentences, and paragraphs. Created documents should be readily identifiable and accessible through electronic filing. It should be easy to store and recall multiple formats, including tabulations and margins. The program should be able to perform complex operations, including the assembly of multiple documents and the production of boilerplate letters to be merged with word processing or data base variables. Boilerplate and other merge functions are critical for a medical practice. They support intricate and automatic written correspondence to patients and referral sources. There are other helpful features such as user-defined keys and print commands. Defined keys can be used to produce words and phrases on a single keystroke. Print commands may include text justification (so that printed material has even right and left margins), roll to top (a command that instructs the printer to roll to the top of the page and is useful in producing multicolumnar copy), super- and subscript, underlining, boldface, and accent marks such as the circumflex (^) and the tilde (~).

Two word processing concepts with which you should be familiar are the Window and the Menu. The Window refers to what you see on the screen as opposed to what is printed. In some word processing programs, the two are not identical. For example, in some programs that call for boldface, boldface is actually shown on the screen. But in other programs, boldface is indicated on the screen by a graphic character before and after the material that will be printed in boldface. The graphic character is not printed but only shows in the screen. This also applies to super-script, underlining, and so on. Because print codes are not a regular part of most MOS word processing, the Window concept is not critical. In any case, most of the people involved in word processing quickly get used to a double-windowed program.

The Menu concept has to do with how convenient a word processing program will be to run and how much training it will take to become proficient with it. A good program will provide quick access to helpful information while it is up and running. It will do this by allowing you to call upon various help menus: menus that will either provide you with information and prompts or actually lead you through the necessary steps. Most important, however, is that the program contain some logic in getting from one place to another.

ADDITIONAL WORD PROCESSING SOFTWARE

There are two add-on word processing software items that are fun and very useful but not essential. These are the spelling and grammar checking programs. The spelling checks will compare each word used in a text against the program's own list of words. If the word is not found, it is flagged or highlighted for user modification. The grammar checks will call attention to word redundancy, the misuse of tense and parallel forms, and violations of other major "rules" of writing. The usefulness of the spelling checks will depend on the number of words in the program's dictionary. Obviously, a 150,000-word dictionary will produce fewer false positives than a 25,000-word dictionary. The dictionary should have a user list so that frequently used specialized words or terms may be added.

GENERAL LEDGER

Relatively inexpensive software is available to help the practitioner with bookkeeping. General ledger programs can assist the practitioner in producing an accurate, easy-to-balance, double-entry system. General ledger programs will provide for a user-defined chart of accounts and user-defined account numbers. In addition, it is important to have automatic features for out-of-balance detection, entry totaling, and document balancing. Ease of document correction, error recovery, and the presentation of well-defined audit trails are important. An error protection control and visually oriented editing are helpful in preventing errant data entry. The following report formats are essential:

a. Chart of accounts.
b. Trial balance.
c. Document list.
d. Posting summary.
e. Ledger detail report.
f. Income statement (profit and loss statement).
g. Balance sheet.

DATA BASE MANAGEMENT

The software for data base systems can be nearly as expensive as word processing packages. Because a good MOS may already have important features of data base management incorporated into it, it is not always necessary for the practitioner to acquire data base management system (DBS) software as an add-on.

The DBS is an electronic "card filing system" that can review the data on various "cards," collate and calculate the data, and present it in formats designated by the user. The simplest use of a

Chapter 3

DBS might be to generate a mailing list. Each file consists of the names and addresses of patients, vendors, friends, and so on. The formats might provide for label or envelope printing to be sorted by zip codes or affiliation. A good DBS will interact with the word processing program to produce multiple, personalized letters.

The DBS has two distinct aspects. One is the creation of the data base, along with its report formats. The other is the utilization of the data base. Utilization is often easy, as the programs are menu driven. Once a mailing list has been set up, for example, all one needs to do is press a key for "label printing" and the rest of the instructions will be delivered by the computer from a series of menus. Setting up the data base for the various report programs is usually much more complicated, and these programs are of the "use it or lose it" variety. The expression "use it or lose it" refers to programs whose commands are so idiosyncratic that unless you are involved with the programs on a daily basis, the commands are likely to be forgotten. Such programs are by no means impossible to set up, but in order to do this the practitioner will either have to take a course or resign herself to careful and tedious study of the manual. The following account is provided by a urologist.

> I had taken a one-day course in data base management, and several weeks later I embarked on creating my own data base. Even in the few weeks that had transpired, I found I had forgotten enough so that it was necessary for me to go back and forth to the manual. My goal was to set up a data base called Super File. In it I planned to include the names and addresses of all people whom I came in contact with, including patients and vendors. In it I would identify variables such as these: Was the person a referral source? Would the person be on a Christmas list? What was the person's nickname or the spouse's name? With it I planned to generate a number of labeling formats as well as formats for dunning, tracking referral sources, and developing a master telephone list. Working two solid weekends, plus mornings and afternoons, it took about two weeks to complete. The problem was that every step of the way I had to check the manual and verify what I did. I had made errors that required redoing several sections. The final product was very satisfactory, and I use it to this day.
>
> A few weeks later, a discussion with my partner resulted in the need to examine the relative length and cost of treatment of each one of our patients. Within a half hour, I was able to produce a new data base, including screen and written formats. This new data base was

no less complicated than the first, and in fact it required the inclusion of statistical variables. The only difference was in my familiarity with the program.

Of course, the practitioner can purchase the program and have a consultant develop the specific data base variables. In terms of cost efficiency, the above practitioner would have been better off if he had had a consultant do this for him on the first go. However, because of the knowledge he gained from his difficult first pass with the program, he became as adept as any consultant who might create data bases for him.

ACCOUNTS PAYABLE AND PAYROLL SYSTEMS

Accounts payable and payroll programs are linked to check-writing procedures and are usually reserved for large practices with large payrolls and unwieldy payables. Do you remember the stories that insurance companies gave you about the computer messing up your check? If you invest in these programs you can be a bona fide user of the same excuse. Generally, such programs are not practical for small operations. It is critical that an accounts payable program be compatible with either a cash or accrual accounting method and that there be relative ease in maintaining accounts. In addition, the following report formats are helpful.

a. Vendor listing.
b. Invoice listing.
c. Posting report with general ledger totals.
d. General ledger recap.
e. Cash requirements.
f. Aging report.
g. Check print.
h. Each check register.
i. Discount loss report.
j. General ledger totals after check printing.

It is helpful if the program prints checks that are suitable for mailing. It is essential that the system be interactive with the general ledger. Otherwise, the system's efficiency is greatly reduced.

Payroll programs should of course, be able to calculate and print all payroll checks. To do so, they must be able to calculate all federal, state, and city payroll taxes. They should be able to print W–2 forms and modified W–2 forms. User-defined categories and classifications for earnings, deductions, and workers' compensation are important, as are automatic voluntary deductions such as savings and insurance. Also important are (1) ease of error correction and recovery and (2) automatic production of a check register and out-of-balance detection. Finally, the system should be interactive with the general ledger.

COMMUNICATION SOFTWARE

The software to communicate with other computers is usually inexpensive (under $30); it's the equipment and royalties that can mount up. The software permits you to link into external data bases (EDB) such as the Dow Jones News Retrieval Service and CompuServe. In this way, your computer becomes a "dumb terminal" using the vast power of a mainframe in Ohio, the District of Columbia, or elsewhere. Each EDB has its own entry codes, passwords, and menus, which you receive when you sign up (and pay up). Chapter 4 is devoted to EDB.

ELECTRONIC SPREAD SHEETS

Supposedly it was an electronic spread sheet, VisiCalc, that made Apple so popular. Electronic spread sheets are fascinating, but not absolutely necessary for a medical practice. A spread sheet, whether mechanical or electronic, looks like the type of balance sheet that an accountant provides. It has a series of vertical and horizontal titles (the months of the year, a list of accounts, etc). In an electronic spread sheet, however, calculation formulas are invisibly placed at various coordinates. Calculations then occur automatically for figures placed on the spread sheet. A potent feature of such programs is that they enable the practitioner to ask "what if" this or that happens to the practice. Looking at the tax liability figure, the practitioner might plug in income and expense information and ask, "What will happen if I see three more patients a week?" Within a few seconds hundreds of figures are recalculated and the answer or answers are revealed on the cathode ray tube (CRT).

Some practitioners use VisiCalc to balance their day sheets and to keep tabs on monthly and quarterly charges, payments, and accounts receivable. Clarity of documentation is particularly important in working electronic spread sheets. New developments have made electronic spread sheets easier to use (through the continuous display of menu choices) and interactive with one another.

ACCOUNTS RECEIVABLE

The accounts receivable program is always part of an MOS. It would not be purchased separately unless the practitioner were putting together her own MOS package or also running a non-medical practice. If you choose to purchase a separate accounts receivable package (perhaps you are putting together your own MOS), then the following requirements should be met. As with all financial packages, it is important that your accounts receivable program be interactive with the general ledger. It is also important that the program be able to define aging and past-due periods and to produce reports of cumulative "sales."

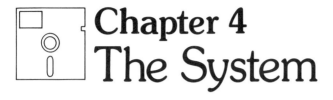

Chapter 4
The System

THE SYSTEM
KEYBOARD
    Configuration
    Feel
    Detachability
CPU
MEMORY AND STORAGE
    Disk Drives
        Floppy Disk Drives
        Hard Disk Drives
    How Much Storage Do You Need?
PRINTER
PRINTERS FOR THE MEDICAL OFFICE
VIDEO DISPLAY
    Radiation
COMMUNICATION HARDWARE
OTHER ITEMS
    Blank Diskettes
    Storage Boxes
    Cables
    Maintenance and Cleaning Supplies
    Antistatic Supplies and Equipment
    Dustcovers
    Power Line Protectors
    Printer Tractor
    Printer Table
    Computer Table
    Fanfold Folders
    Data Racks
    Print Ruler
    Labels and Felt Tip Pens
    Data Trays

THE SYSTEM

Most readers of this book will already have some knowledge about the basic hardware configuration of a computer system. To review this subject briefly, there are essentially five elements in a professional office computer system: (1) keyboard (for input), (2) microprocessor (CPU, or central processing unit) and volatile storage medium (both configured together and sometimes referred to as the computer), (3) disk drive (storage medium), (4) output devices (video display, or CRT, and printer), and (5) modem (communication hardware). In the following sections the components of all five elements are discussed, with detail given regarding applicability to a medical, dental, or psychological office.

KEYBOARD

Configuration

The simplest computer keyboard resembles a typewriter keyboard. It has the 26 letters of the alphabet; numbers 0–9; punctuation and other symbols, including plus and minus signs; and two or more command keys, including the shift and enter keys. More sophisticated keyboards house program- and system-related keys, the most common of which is the break key. This key will halt the operation of a program written in BASIC, permitting various types of user intervention. It may also be used, depending on the program and language, to move in reverse along a menu pattern. (For details about menus, refer to Chapter 8.) A caps key is used to capitalize all alphabetic characters without affecting numeric ones. When the operator is working with a large group of capitalized letters, this key avoids the tedium of having to continually use the shift key while going back and forth from numbers to letters. There may also be keys labeled tab, hold, repeat, control, and escape. These command keys will take on properties designated by particular programs. The keyboard may also have function keys, usually labeled F1, F2, F3, and so on. These keys may be used by a program either to perform specific functions while working at a given menu level or to move the user from one menu level to another. For example, in some word processing programs the F2 key is used in a way that makes the cursor appear to gobble up the letters like Pac-Man. Keeping the F2 and repeat keys down for about 30 seconds would be enough to wipe out almost anybody's correspondence. Usually the F2 key is used only to obliterate an errant letter or word. In a general ledger program the F2 key may be used to "Exit to the main menu." However, the array of functions keys has little value without a program for using them. In other words, if your programs use only F1 and F2, having F3–F9 on the keyboard will make it look more fancy but will have no immediate value.

A numeric pad is a convenience. This is an extra set of numeric keys configured like a calculator and usually set off to the right of the keyboard. Another convenience is to have the add, subtract, multiply, and divide signs placed on the pad, rather than hidden among the standard keys.

The relative position and size of certain keys, particularly the break key, can be important. Programs written in BASIC are particularly vulnerable to unintentional use of the break key, which might obliterate all the information on your screen at that time.

There are keyboards with every conceivable configuration of alphanumeric keys, function keys, and control keys. These keys are often "captured by a program" and are meant to make the system more "user friendly." For example, if the keyboard has a key labeled print, the operator would press it instead of pressing the control and P keys simultaneously. Pressing this one key does what might otherwise take two or three keys to do. However, apart from saving the user from having to memorize combination keystrokes, such added keys serve no great need.

Feel

Some keyboards feel as if they were sculpted by a craftsperson, others as if they came out of a plastic punch machine. To date, there is no study showing that, after the first few days of use, one type of keyboard increases or decreases productivity or that the owner or operator cares anymore. It is unlikely that any reader of this book will plan to run a practice with a pocket computer. It's probably safe to say that any keyboard will feel OK if it comes with a computer that is going to run the programs referred to in this book. There are so many opportunities to agonize about the variables among computer systems that this variable should be put close to the bottom of the list.

Detachability

In *The Word Processing Book* Peter McWilliams emphasizes the importance of the detachability of the keyboard from the computer console so that, for example, the keyboard might be placed on your lap. The keyboard is attached to the CPU only by cable.[1] McWilliams feels so strongly about this that he will not recommend a computer for word processing if the keyboard is not detachable.

> A practitioner in Utah writes:
>
> After reading McWilliams book, I asked, "How could someone who knows so much about computers be wrong?" So, my computer has a detachable keyboard. And I also learned what Mr. McWilliams meant when he said that just because he preferred something didn't mean that all his readers would.
>
> My secretary had no interest in having a keyboard in any other position than attached directly to the computer. Being a pioneer, I attempted to demonstrate to her the convenience of placing the keyboard in my lap. One of the first things that happened was that a pencil fell out of my ear and dropped on the break key while I was in a BASIC program, resulting in a minor disaster. Undaunted, I persisted, but to sit in one of those laid-back positions you see on TV or in magazine ads, you either have to face away from the screen or be far enough away from it to need binoculars to read the material.
>
> In my office the keyboard now rests abutted to the computer. It might as well be attached by steel beams.

Despite the example given above, there are a number of good reasons for having a detachable keyboard. Any ability that the operator has to adjust the surroundings tends to increase the potential for comfort. A slight variation in the position of the keyboard, even one inch, might lend to an improved angle of view or a reduction in glare. Occasionally, the keyboard becomes the control panel for operating the printer. Being able to place the keyboard adjacent to the printer for such special operations may be a real convenience. And finally, having a detachable keyboard would certainly facilitate repair of the keyboard if it were the only

---

[1] Recent developments now permit complete detachment of the keyboard. Messages are sent from it to the computer via radio frequency waves.

element that needed to be serviced. It is easier to bring the keyboard in for service than an entire computer.

CPU

When this book was being written, the 16-bit personal computer had begun to establish itself on the market. For the average doctor, however, it doesn't matter whether the computer is 8 bits or 16 bits. For the uninitiated, bytes refer to the size of the electronic words that the computer can use to conduct its affairs. Some computers use 8-bit words (8-bit bytes, so to speak); others use 16-bit words. To understand the relevance of this feature, think of a dump truck carrying cords of wood. If you have lots of wood to haul, obviously a 16-cord truck is going to be better than an 8-cord truck. Each trip will net a bigger payload. But what if your workers or equipment were "programmed" to load only eight cords at a time, no matter what the size of the truck. You would end up having a lot more truck than you could use. So it is with computers. Although the 16-bit and 16/32-bit computer may be the hallmark of the future, at present most of the tested medically oriented software is written for the 8-bit microprocessor. To deal with this discrepancy, most 16-bit computers come with an 8-bit microprocessor. The added expense of a 16-bit microprocessor will be worthwhile only if all your programs are written for it. There may be difficulty in switching back and forth from 8-bit programs to 16-bit programs. If you are using a hard disk drive, it will be impossible. This means that the doctor would need to have all programs written in 16 bits to get full and efficient use out of a 16-bit computer.

Most 8-bit business microcomputers are constructed so that they can be upgraded to a 16-bit computer. So the conversion can occur if absolutely necessary. Unfortunately, there is no guarantee that data stored in an 8-bit program can be transferred to a 16-bit program. Transfer from an 8-bit program to a 16-bit program might mean entering data from scratch. Most practitioners who have already gone through the process of setting up a computerized MOS would not willingly do it again.

In brief, if you are able to find an array of medical practice software written for a 16-bit computer, then you will have a system that will work faster and more efficiently. If the software you choose is configured for an 8-bit CPU, then the venture into a 16-bit operation will be superfluous.

MEMORY AND STORAGE

Memory is most often referred to as RAM, random access memory. RAM is volatile memory that is needed to run and use a program at any given moment. It is lost once the computer is turned off. Memory sounds like storage, but in computerese the terms *storage* and *memory* have different meanings. To understand the difference between RAM and storage, let's use a football analogy. Storage refers to the size of the playbook—to the number of plays that might be indexed in one playbook. RAM refers to the number of plays that the coach and team can remember at any given moment without looking back at the playbook.

Let's say that the Detroit Lions can remember only two plays at a time (small RAM) but that their playbook holds a thousand different plays (large disk storage). Although they have many plays to look up, they can remember only two. They can, therefore, compare the relative worth of only one play against another. To compare more plays, they would have to go back to the playbook and look up another two; but in so doing, they forget the first two.

The New England Patriots, on the other hand, are able to remember and compare 100 plays at any given moment (large RAM), but their tiny playbook holds only a maximum of 10 plays (small disk storage). They can compare these 10 plays with lightning speed, but that's it—they can't compare more plays than they have in one playbook.

Most eight-bit programs require at least 64K of RAM (64,000 bytes of random access memory). Sixteen-bit multi-user operations (more about that in Chapter 15) may require from 125K to 750K of RAM. For most eight-bit single-user MOS operations, 80K of RAM is probably adequate. Storage is another matter.

Disk Drives

Long-term storage, that is, information stored between uses of the computer, is most commonly done on disk drives. At the time of writing, developments in alternative storage media were steadily coming forth. Nonetheless, it's probably safe to say that disk drives will be as common on the computer scene as tape recorders have been on the music scene. There may be variations, but the essential principles and equipment will endure. The choice then lies between hard disk and floppy disk; and then among the various sizes and configurations within these groups. Most readers will know the difference between floppy disk and hard disk. The following explanation is practical, not technical (like an explanation that says a carburetor mixes air and fuel rather than telling precisely how this is done).

Hard disk drives store about 8 to 20 times as much information per drive as floppy disks. They cost from three to five times as much. In 90 percent of hard disk drives the storage medium is sealed and not user removable, whereas floppy disks may be inserted and removed at will. Typically, separate programs are stored on different floppy disks. So if you want to run word processing, you put in the word processing disk. (The data that you store is often kept on the same disk as the program.) If you then want to switch to general ledger, you take out the word processing disk and you put in the general ledger disk. In a sense, floppy disk drives can "store" an infinite amount of information; that is, the amount of storage is limited only by one's library of floppy disks. However, putting in and taking out diskettes is more laborious than the uninitiated might think. Every program has an entry and exit procedure, and the entire process may take several minutes. Multiply that by 20 switches a day, and an hour a day can be wasted. Moreover, this method does not facilitate disk interaction or global searches across diskettes.

Floppy Disk Drives. Floppy diskettes got their name because that's what they are—floppy. They are either 5½- or 8-inch platters consisting of essentially the same material with which cassette tapes are made. They are somewhat permanently housed in sealed envelopes with a sliver exposed, just enough for a magnetic head to "read" and "write" on the disk. They are designed to be inserted and removed from disk drives just as tape cartridges are inserted and removed from an eight-track stereo. Hard disks, on the other hand, are rigid platters, almost always sealed within the disk drive itself and not usually designed to be inserted or removed by the user.

Enter multiple disk drives. One of the solutions to the problem of switching diskettes is to have a bank of floppy disk drives, with the first drive serving as a controller for all the attached drives. The MOS is placed in the first drive (some systems refer to this as Drive 0). General ledger, word processing, and other programs are placed in "secondary drives." Notwithstanding programming conflicts, the user can quickly switch from one drive to another, one program to another—can even merge programs—without the inconvenience of physically putting in and removing disks.

Hard Disk Drives. Sometimes referred to as a Winchester disk drive (faster than a speeding bullet), the hard disk drive works about 10 times as fast as floppy. One hard disk drive may contain several platters. But no matter what the internal mechanisms of the hard disk drive, it is referred to in a way that would imply that it contains only one platter. Because the storage capacity of the hard disk drive is so great (3 to 15 million bytes per drive), a number of obvious advantages occur:

1. Many programs, ranging from accounts receivable to word processing, may stored on the same drive.
2. Considerable data may be stored and indexed on a single drive.
3. Access time is reduced both because it is not necessary to swap disks and because mechanically hard disk systems operate at faster speeds.

Like floppy disks, hard disks can be placed together in a configuration of primary and secondary drives.

Practitioners who switch from floppy to hard disk expecting to upgrade to a lightning-fast operation are invariably disappointed. Such practitioners may expect the hard disk system to respond instantaneously, information to appear on keystroke. But nothing is as fast as RAM. Disk drives may approach the speed of sound, but RAM approaches the speed of light. No mechanical maneuver will be as fast as an electronic one. In the not too distant future, bubble memory and "disk" RAM will start to bridge this gap.

There are two time-consuming aspects of any type of disk memory transfer to RAM: (1) Some programs call for the passing of parameters or information among several files. Although this may be done rather rapidly, it still takes time—10 or more seconds in some programs. (2) It also takes time for the information to be loaded from the hard disk drive to the computer (CPU). Information is passed in series; that is, one bit follows another. For lengthy and complex programs, the wait may seem unnecessarily long to the impatient. Many hard disk drives are advertised as being 5 to 10 times faster than floppy, but this refers to the searching mechanism. For example, Profile is a versatile, easy-to-use data base management program. What is invisible to the user is that its internal layout is very complex. The most frequently used menu item is one called "Inquire, update, review." In floppy it takes about 40 seconds to get into this mode. In a hard disk it takes 10 seconds less, but that is still a 30-second wait. Hard disk is indeed faster than floppy, but there is still a lot of finger tapping going on while the program is coming around.

There are, however, other advantages to hard disk drives. Besides operating faster, hard disk drives differ from floppy on two other variables: (1) they have a larger storage capacity—usually about 20 times as large as that of floppy disk; (2) the operating system requires proportionately less space on the disk. The operating system refers to about 18–20 files used by the computer company to tell the CPU and disk drives how to work. The computer cannot do anything worthwhile without it. When you use floppy disks, this system must be recorded on every disk used in the first drive. If you have programs on 10 different floppy disks, then you also have 10 copies of the operating system taking up space. In a hard disk operation, these 18–20 files appear only once.

To simplify the mysteries and wonder of hard disk, one might visualize it as operating like one huge floppy disk. On it is placed a copy of the operating system plus each program (word processing, MOS, etc.), with lots of space left over to record data and updates. Because everything is on one disk, compatible programs can be interrelated with great facility. Moreover, with hard disk it is easy to develop *user* menus, that is, menus and routines created by the doctor himself.

The above advantages of hard disk—large storage capacity, no physical manipulation of disks, potential for interrelating programs, and ease of creating user menus—make it much more user friendly than floppy disk. For example, the following master menu might be brought up automatically when a hard disk operation is first turned on in the morning:

1. Medical Office System.
2. Word processing.
3. Financial spread sheets.
4. Data base management.
5. Dow Jones News Retrieval Service.
6. Printing.

Pressing option 6 (printing) might bring up this printing submenu, also created by the doctor:

1. Envelope (title, first, last name).
2. Envelope (as above, with position and company name).
3. Label (title, first and last name).

In hard disk operations it is easy to type an envelope of someone on file. There is no loading of special disks. At the main menu the secretary need only press option 6, then option 1 or 2; answer a prompt as to the name of the individual to be retrieved; put an envelope in the printer; and press the enter key. The job will probably be complete before she has a chance to look from the keyboard to the printer.

How Much Storage Do You Need?

The two largest presses on storage space come from the financial aspects of the MOS and from word processing. If you plan to store all correspondence and patient progress notes on an electronic medium, you will need a storage capacity that may defy imagination. Most word processing storage occurs in ASCII, a coding system that gobbles up available data bits at an alarmingly fast rate. The following guidelines may be helpful in determining what kind of storage capacity you will need.

Most MOS application programs use up from 200K to 300K bytes. That in itself is about the average space of an 8-inch double-density, single-sided disk. In addition to this, you will need from 1K to 2K bytes for each patient stored on the system (active or inactive). Word processing, general ledger, data base management and electronic spread sheet program files may each occupy 50K to 200K bytes of storage. For word processing, 1K–2K bytes will be needed to store each 250–500-word page. Electronic spread sheets require 1K–18K bytes for each "sheet" stored. With these figures it is not difficult to see how 10 million bytes of storage will soon be needed by a medium-sized, single-practitioner office.

The typical practice of 100 patient contact hours per week will press two floppy disk drives to their limits. Psychological/psychiatric practices, even those with multiple therapists, may be run on two disk drives without major difficulty. This is because of relatively slow turnover. In such practices one patient may be seen for 50 hours rather than 50 patients for one hour.

An assumption is made that after 30–90 days invoices that have been zeroed out by payment or adjustment will be hard-copied and purged from the system, leaving space for fresh data. If the practitioner wishes to keep such archives in the microcomputer, then storage will need to be doubled or tripled, depending on how long the archives are kept.

If it is apparent that more than two floppy disk drives will be needed, then consideration should be given to an initial investment in a hard disk drive. Most practices which will be using interactive programs (financial and word processing) will benefit from the added convenience and speed of such a drive.

PRINTER

The printer and video display are the only two output devices likely to be used in an MOS. In this book, printers will be referred to as though there were only two types: dot matrix and Daisy Wheel. There are other types, but why make things complicated? Dot matrix printers form characters by printing a matrix of tiny dots, usually five across and seven down per character. The larger the matrix (7 by 9 instead of 5 by 7, for example), the sharper the characters and the greater the expense of the printer. Dot matrix printers are almost always faster than Daisy Wheel printers, printing from 500 to 3,000 words a minute, yet they will be within the average user's budget. However, regardless of the size of the matrix and the method of imprinting the character on the paper, dot matrix printers do not have the Selectric typewriter look that Daisy Wheel printers produce.

Everyone knows about the element (ball) in the IBM Selectric that spins around and goes back and forth, printing words on the page. The Daisy Wheel is a variant of that element. Given instructions from the printer, it places a crisp character on the paper. The

Daisy Wheel itself is prone to wear and injury, but it is easy to replace and it costs less than $40. Daisy Wheel printers produce crisp, letter-quality correspondence, but at a price. They are slower than dot matrix printers, with the usual affordable machine producing between 100 and 500 words a minute. The faster the Daisy Wheel printer, the more expensive it is. In addition, most Daisy Wheel printers are noisy little buggers. The Daisy Wheel's decibel level is about 60, which Judy Graf Klein's *The Office Book* de-

FIGURE 4–1
Printer*

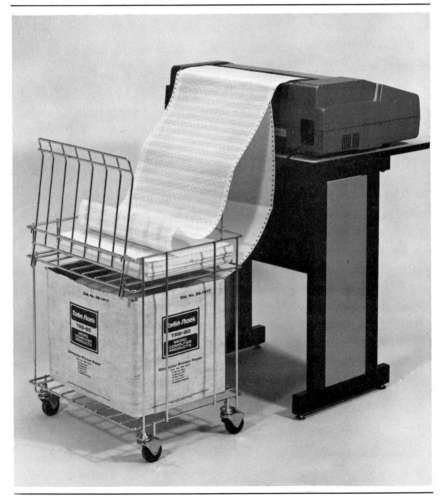

* Permission to reprint given by Radio Shack, a division of the Tandy Corporation.

scribes as in the range of a "congested department store." The sound from the printer is continuous and not unpleasant when the Daisy Wheel is doing a run. However, you will be unable to have a telephone conversation within 10 feet of it without putting a finger in your other ear. There is often a slight motion or vibration as the Daisy Wheel flies back and forth. One gets the feeling that there's enough hydraulic force within this tiny machine to lift a car eight feet off the ground. Most Daisy Wheel printers can vibrate the screws and legs out of a flimsy table within a week or two. More about this in the section on computer furniture.

Within the last year, dot matrix printers that produce letter-quality copy have been introduced. When you look at the results, you will say, "That's amazing; I can hardly tell the difference." In other words, the finished product of the new dot matrix printers is *almost* as good as that of the Daisy Wheel. They are fast, upward of 3,000 words per minute, and they cost about as much as a 500-word-per-minute Daisy Wheel printer.

All printers require more office space than the novice user would expect (see Figure 4-1). In addition to the room needed for the table on which the printer is placed, if continuous forms are used, there must be room to store the pile of forms going in and the pile coming out. Access to the front of the printer is needed so that controls can be set or text checked, and at least three feet of space is needed in back of it to collect printed matter on a caddy or an attached bin. Bottom fed printers require less space.

PRINTERS FOR THE MEDICAL OFFICE

Unless you are going to buy two printers, which is somewhat impractical (not only does this cost more, but they take up a lot of space), you will need to choose between a dot matrix printer and a Daisy Wheel printer. The principal determinant will be whether or not letter-quality correspondence and reports must be produced. If the answer is yes, then buy the fastest Daisy Wheel printer you can afford. However, any Daisy Wheel printer that is slower than 500 words a minute (about 43 cps) is likely to be a disappointment. This rate may seem fast, but when a 500-wpm printer is applied to, say, insurance forms, it will take from 30 to 60 seconds to print a form. There may not be 500 words to be typed on an insurance form, but because the Daisy Wheel must travel completely from the left to the right margin and complete its cycle, it may act as though there were. This means that the printer might take from one to two hours to print 100 insurance forms. The same difficulty arises in connection with financial reports and patient statements.

If your practice can get by with *nearly* letter-quality correspondence, then you should consider one of the faster, crisper dot matrix printers. A 3,000-wpm dot matrix printer could polish off 100 insurance forms in 10 to 20 minutes.

Because carbon copies of both correspondence and insurance forms are often required in a medical practice, the printing must be done by impact rather than jet ink or electrical burning.

If you are producing more than 15 pages of correspondence and 30 pages of report forms daily, including insurance and patient statements, then consider purchasing both a dot matrix printer and a Daisy Wheel printer. However, such volume usually indicates that a multi-user system is required. This special computer configuration is discussed in Chapter 15.

VIDEO DISPLAY

The video display (or CRT—cathode-ray tube) is probably a more important factor in user comfort and productivity than are the keyboard configuration and feel. The standard for commercial use is a video display of 80 characters across and 24 down and a 12-inch screen (measured diagonally). Anything less will compromise comfort and productivity. Also, the smaller the matrix of the screen, the more frequently must the user scroll either horizontally or vertically to view the work. Although one can eke out correspondence on a screen 64 characters across, viewing financial readouts can be quite cumbersome. Some monitors have an 80 by 50 matrix, permitting full view of the page. This is an obvious convenience, but such monitors cost more than twice as much as conventional monitors.

Crispness or clarity of the image is very important. Green phosphorus monitors produce high resolution and are recommended. The traditional black-and-white TV tube delivers a slightly fuzzy image, which is OK for watching a movie but is likely to cause eyestrain after about 15 minutes of close contact. Keep in mind that the operator may be expected to stare at that screen for hours a day at a distance that our parents told us would make our eyes go bad.

Radiation

Not a great deal has been published regarding the amount of radiation absorbed by computer operators sitting in front of the CRT.[2] Most studies show that the amount falls substantially within currently acceptable levels. There is some equivocal evidence that emitted microwaves may produce eye problems. Until the evidence is clear, periodic eye examinations would be recommended for those looking at a CRT for more than 20 hours a week.

COMMUNICATION HARDWARE

Modem (an acronym for Modulation-Demodulation unit) permits computers to communicate over telephone lines. The prices of these units range from $100 to $1,200 and vary according to automatic features and the baud rate (the rate of speed at which the modem can receive and transmit). The most common quality-constructed modem costs about $150, transmits at a rate of 300 baud, and requires user manipulation to start and stop computer transmission or reception. This piece of communication equipment is essential for linkage to external data bases, such as the Dow Jones News Retrieval Service and MEDLAR. When using external data bases, the user is charged by the hour. Because communication may involve long-distance phone calls or tariffed access lines, frequent and prolonged use of this telecommunication route would warrant investment in a more expensive—1,200 baud—modem. Not to be outdone, most data base companies will charge a higher rate for higher baud communication. More about this in Chapter 13. For the doctor who wishes to dabble with data bases and other telecommunication routes, a modem such as the Radio Shack Direct Connect I is recommended. It sells for about $100. The computer must also have an RS-232 interface and port which is standard on most models costing more than $2,000.

---

[2] L. Slesin and M. Zybko, "VDT's: Health and Safety," excerpts from *Microwave News*, 1983.

OTHER ITEMS

Before you become a full-fledged microcomputer user, you may have the illusion that investment in the above items is sufficient to get a system going. It isn't. You'll find that the items listed below are either necessary or helpful.

Blank Diskettes

Floppy disk drive users will need 30 to 40 extra disks to start and will have to figure on adding about 20 disks a year. These will be used to make backups of application programs and daily, weekly, or monthly data saves. Hard disk drive users will need about half this amount, unless backups are made on tape. If the latter is the case, a half-dozen floppies may be needed for miscellaneous use.

Storage Boxes

Floppy users will need five small storage boxes and one large one. The large box will be labeled "Today" and will house all disks to be used currently. Of the five small boxes, one will house the originals of all the application programs (and be put in a safe). The remaining three will be marked A, B, and C and will store the rotation of backups. (More about this in Chapter 6.) The fifth box will be used for monthly or yearly saves.

If the hard disk drive is backed up to floppy disks, the user will need three small boxes—one for original application floppy disks, one for daily or weekly saves, and the third for monthly or yearly saves.

Cables

A cable connecting the printer to the computer is not normally thought of as an integral part of either the printer or the computer; at least, not as any more integral than speaker wire is to an amplifier and speaker. When you buy any equipment that is to be attached to the computer, do not assume that the cable comes with it. Unfortunately, different computers require different cable configurations; there is no industry standard.

One psychologist who had been looking forward to entering the world of telecomputing communication was very excited when her modem finally arrived. But she then had to cool her heels because she had not ordered the cable. Cable costs vary with the complexity and length of the cable. Most 6-foot cables cost about $30.

Maintenance and Cleaning Supplies

The accessible parts of floppy disk drives and Daisy Wheel printers require cleaning. Both the magnetic head of the disk drive and the Daisy Wheels themselves will accumulate debris (especially if the printer uses an inked ribbon). The necessary cleaning supplies and equipment are readily available and will cost a total of less than $40.

Antistatic Supplies and Equipment

Static electricity can generate 10,000–50,000 volts of low-amperage electricity and is capable of wiping out the RAM contents or a sector of a disk. A conductive antistatic mat, attached to an electrical ground, may be placed in the immediate area under and around the computer. It drains static charges from users. Another antistatic device is a relatively inexpensive spray, available at most computer stores. It may be applied monthly to the carpet and other areas that are likely to generate static electricity. Mats cost about $75; sprays about $5.

Dustcovers

Although these may be the most inexpensive items purchased, they are the most critical in terms of computer care. Dust will eventually gum up the keyboard, clog or ruin disk drives, and generally do in both floppy and hard disks. The illustration on page 44 is worth a thousand words.

Power Line Protectors

There are many products on the market to protect the computer from sudden reductions or surges in AC power. These power line

Sizes of Common Pollutants

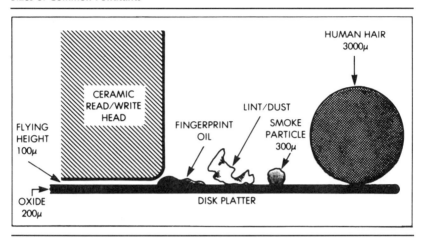

Source: Reprinted with permission from Rodnay Zaks, *Don't! (Or How to Care for Your Computer)* (Berkeley, Calif.: SYBEX, Inc., 1981).

protectors may be combined with a nickel-cadmium battery and rectifier to produce temporary alternating current during a total power loss. The current is usually supplied for a short time, but long enough to permit the user to close the system down in a stepwise fashion, thus protecting data. Frequently, line protectors are configured with four to six female plugs and may be designed so that all peripherals are plugged into outlets that are turned on and off automatically when the computer is turned on and off. A good line protector with six female plugs, five of which are automatically linked to the on/off switch of the computer, can be purchased for under $80. It is recommended for three reasons: (1) it reduces the mess of extension cord wires; (2) it saves time in powering up and powering down the system; and (3) it provides some protection against line voltage variance. Line protectors that produce alternative power cost over $500 and are just not cost efficient for the average practitioner. An adequate backup routine will take care of minor floppy and hard disk crashes should the "lights go off."

Printer Tractor

Unless it is an integral part of a printer, a tractor will need to be purchased for a medical practice. Without a tractor, paper is fed through the printer by friction, the platen pressing against other rollers and the paper wedged in between. This method is common to all conventional typewriters, and it works fine if you are feeding and lining up each sheet individually. However, if the alignment is off 1/100 inch on a run of 100 continuous insurance forms or statements, the last form will be printed an inch out of alignment. Once the tractor is in place, the platen may be adjusted so that the paper is moved along by sprockets on the tractor rather than the friction of the platen. The sprockets fit into the little holes along the sides of green bar or other continuous-run forms. Alignment is absolutely precise. A tractor costs about $200.

Printer Table

A special table is needed for the printer. If you have a bottom-fed printer, it will require a table with a slot cut to accept paper from beneath. Special places are needed to which bins for the collection of fanfold printouts may be attached. Paper feeding and collection are hindered by the excessive depth of a standard table. And finally, because most Daisy Wheel printers vibrate, the table must be solidly and thoughtfully constructed. Daisy Wheel printers should not be placed on the same table as computers or any other equipment that would be adversely affected by vibration.

Computer Table

The type of computer you have will influence the type of table you need for it. A console requires a well-constructed table or desk that is about typing height (28 inches). Computer systems that have separate components (disk drives, CRT, and keyboard) are sometimes best served by a multilevel desk. A built-in drawer is helpful. Otherwise, the only considerations would be aesthetic. Some users like to have the computer desk compatible in design with the printer table. White desks are modern looking, but they may contribute to eyestrain (see Chapter 9).

Fanfold Folders

Unburst green bar (computer paper with the pin holes in the margins) is unwieldy to handle unless it is placed in special folders. These folders are constructed so that the user can flip through the pages of green bar with ease. The folders hold 500–1,000 pages and may be used to consolidate reports on: accounts receivable, daily recap, transactions and patient diagnostic and procedure data.

Data Racks

Because fanfold folders are large and cumbersome, they are best housed in a special rack. A typical rack can hold up to 12 folders with as many as 400 pages of green bar in each folder.

Print Ruler

This $2.89 item is essential in the drafting of report formats. In addition to being marked by inches, the print ruler is marked to measure 10 and 12-pitch characters horizontally across the page, as well as number and position of the lines along the vertical. If your insurance form printing format is user alterable, a print ruler will be necessary to complete the task.

Labels and Felt Tip Pens

Extra labels are affixed to floppy disks when content is changed significantly. Because floppy disks are vulnerable to pressure, felt tip pens are used to write on the labels.

Data Trays

Because most green bar is nearly 15 inches wide, the usual in/out stacking tray will be too narrow for your computer work. There is nothing very special about data trays except that they are at more than 14 inches wide and convenient for computer use.

For a complete listing of all the items needed to make your system operational, go to the end of Chapter 11.

Chapter 5
Starting Up the MOS

TAKE 90 DAYS
WHEN'S THE BEST TIME TO START
TIME REALLOCATION
    Training
    Practice
    Routine Use
THE AGONY OF DEFEAT AND THE ECSTASY
  OF VICTORY
    Previous Accounts
    Quirks in Recording and Amending Transactions
    Learning Systems Commands and Techniques
    Reporting Techniques
    Aging and Dunning Messages
INSURANCE FORMS
ADEQUATE SUPPLIES

TAKE 90 DAYS

Recently, a lawyer told me that he had had a DEC computer for two years and would be attempting to use the accounts receivable package for the first time. He felt it took that long to get comfortable with the word processing and litigation support programs before going on to other programs. Most users will not need that much time to make their systems completely operable, but the message is well taken. It takes a while to learn the system and to get everything going. To expect everything to be running from day one is unrealistic. A more realistic goal is to take up to 90 days to get an MOS going completely, particularly if it is started sometime after February.

WHEN'S THE BEST TIME TO START?

The best time to put an MOS into effect is the beginning of December. That will give you one month of trial runs before you enter January figures. Any system begun after January 1 will need to have figures added retroactively. Consider this. Say you do start the system in January. A patient comes in January 3, and the procedure and transactions are entered into the computer. At the end of the month an insurance form is generated, and perhaps a bill to the patient. Your reporting system includes this transaction and all others in a January report. But what about the patient seen December 15 who hasn't paid yet or whose insurance company hasn't sent a payment? The point is that for a certain period of time it will be necessary to run your old billing system and the computer billing system simultaneously. In most practices it takes about 90 days to turn around the billing system. The alternative is to retroactively enter 90 days' worth of transactions into the computer. This can mean entering anywhere from 2,000 to 5,000 transactions. This process might take two to three weeks. For this reason alone, it is not possible to convert to a completely computerized system overnight. Some retroactive entering will be necessary.

Any system put into effect after January will need to have the year's earlier transactions placed retroactively into the computer if one wishes to use the computer for financial reporting for that year. This may be necessary in practices with partnerships and other business entities that have complicated financial considerations. However, making retroactive entries is such an enormous task, that it is not recommended if the system is put into effect after the first quarter of the year. Rather, it is best to use the system for partial recording of practice activities for the remainder of the year and then put it into full effect on January of the forthcoming year.

TIME REALLOCATION

It will be necessary for operators of the computer to reallocate their time. This applies not only to the secretary but also to the practitioner. The biggest change in time allocation will occur during the first six weeks that the computer is in operation. Then, more time than would ordinarily be needed on an ongoing basis will be used for training and start-up procedures. In general, time will have been allocated for these three purposes: training, practice, and routine use.

Training

It takes time to learn about the computer's operating system and the software involved. This may be accomplished through self-study, consultant tutorials, or formal instruction. Word processing takes about 10 hours of formal instruction; MOS, 10 hours; data base management, 6 hours; and financial spread sheets, 6 hours. Figure on taking three times as long for self-instruction.

Practice

After the instruction has been completed, it will take about three times as many hours to master the various techniques and commands embodied in these programs. For example, it takes about 10 seconds to type in the commands to do a backup (though the backup procedure may take as long as a half hour for the computer to perform). However, the command and procedure require so much precision that many novices will spend hours trying to accomplish their first few backup routines. If it takes 10 hours to be taught a word processing system, figure on an additional 30 hours of work to master it.

Most systems have quirks and special commands that eventually become second nature to the operator. Unfortunately, most programs are of a "use it or lose it" variety. If they are not used with some regularity, the idiosyncratic commands tend to be forgotten. This means going back to the manual when the program is reused.

Routine Use

Eventually, the computer and its programs will become part of the everyday office routine. When this occurs, the allocation of computer time will become more predictable and better planned. Unless yours is a multi-user system, some regulation of computer use may be necessary. Unlike the typewriter which is usually allocated to one staff member, the computer may take on a "universal owner" aura. Regardless of the number of users, computers, or terminals, one person should be in charge of the computer operation and the allocation of computer time.

THE AGONY OF DEFEAT AND THE ECSTASY OF VICTORY

Starting up an MOS is a procedure that provides ample occasions for success and failure. After the initial excitement of getting the equipment, the unprepared user has many opportunities for disappointment. The following situations are given, not as prophecies of doom, but rather as indications of typical problems that practitioners encounter in setting up an MOS.

Previous Accounts

A nearly universal problem is recording previous accounts receivable. Most systems do not have a start-up procedure for recording balances acquired prior to the initial use of the computer. It is therefore necessary to designate a procedure called "Previous balance" as the first entry on the patient's electronic ledger.

Quirks in Recording and Amending Transactions

Every program has idiosyncrasies that will dictate the manner in which financial transactions are recorded and amended. In Chapter 2 it was pointed out that a transaction has many segments. For a charge transaction there are date of service, procedure, diagnosis, geographic location of service, doctor who provided service, responsibility for payment (insurance company or patient), number of times procedure was performed, and charge for procedure. On the payment side of transactions there are date paid, amount paid, payer (insurance company or patient), and adjustments (for example, a write-off). Some programs have features that become "locked in." In some programs, for example, on a given invoice only one physician may be recorded for providing a service. So, if two practitioners see the patient, it would be necessary to produce two invoices. Other programs "lock in" the party responsible for payment (insurance company or patient), making it difficult to switch in midstream.

Learning Systems Commands and Techniques

Although it is unnecessary for the user to learn programming per se, the user has to be familiar with program commands and utility commands. Program commands are often, but not always, generated by menu. Most MOS packages are completely menu driven. However, electronic spread sheets and data base management systems may be only partially menu driven, requiring user familiarity with commands. A command may be as simple as pressing Control Q to quit the program, but the user still has to know that. During the first weeks of setting up, there is often tedious reference to the manual.

Utility commands involve specific aspects of the computer's system. Such commands are sometimes incorporated into a program and are menu driven. For example, many MOS packages have a menu item called "Backup" that will prompt the user through the backup procedure. However, there are numerous commands which are not frequently found in program menus and these include:

1. DIRECTORY. This is used to review the names of files currently on the disk directory.
2. FREE. This is used to determine how much space is left on a disk and, on some programs, what locations on the disk are still free for data entry.
3. ECHO, DUAL, and SCREEN. These are printer commands that permit either simultaneous entry of material on the screen and the printer or a dumping of all the material that is on the screen to the printer.
4. COPY, DELETE, RENAME, and MOVE. These are commands that are used to manipulate disk files.

Reporting Techniques

Most MOS packages require specific events to take place in a specific sequence. It goes without saying that transactions must be entered before they may appear on a patient's statement. But which comes first, daily posting or transaction report, accounts receivable report or monthly billing? Will account aging be tied to the date entered versus the date run, or will it be tied to specific billing procedures? The point is that every system has its own quirks, as the following example illustrates.

One pediatrician meticulously entered his January, February, and March transactions retroactively in April (when he initiated the system) so that he could have a full calendar year of reporting, from January to January. His MOS produced nifty bar graphs giving monthly comparisons of such things as accounts receivable and write-offs. Information was transferred to this bar graph program in a procedure called "Monthly purge." On April 1 the doctor did the purge for March, which seemed logical. Unfortunately, the program was written to place all remaining entries in the present month. Had the doctor "fooled" the computer and said that it was March 31 (instead of April 1), all would have been fine. However, the doctor had inadvertently placed all March figures in April. Also, the doctor and his secretary had decided that backups would be done after the purge. He quickly found that he had bar graphs for January and February, none for March, and double figures for April. Without a backup before the purge, the program was set in concrete, so to speak. Despite the doctor's meticulous efforts to enter figures retroactively, the March and April bar graphs had limited value that year.

Aging and Dunning Messages

Since aging and dunning messages will reflect the time differential between the date the transaction is entered and the date the statement is run, some caution is recommended when performing retroactive entries. In starting up an MOS, one practitioner retroactively entered transactions from March but inadvertently coded statements as though they were being run in February. As a result, accounts were electronically marked as though they were 11 months old. Stern dunning messages were then printed on all the accounts.

Program quirks of this sort can disappoint and frustrate the practitioner. But such errors can often be avoided by meticulously following detailed documentation or the advice of a person who has had experience with a similar program. The practitioner who expects to fly through the setup procedure without a hitch is probably being unrealistic.

INSURANCE FORMS

There may be a greater variety of insurance forms than computers. These forms vary according to the types and categories of information asked and where the specific data are supposed to be placed. Even the so-called standard AMA universal insurance form has revisions. Trying to figure out the differences between forms is like trying to figure out one of those puzzles that asks you to find six differences between two pictures that look identical. The differences in the insurance forms *are* there, and those differences become painfully obvious when information is printed in margins, lines, or headings. If you are unfortunate enough to have an MOS that lacks a user-alterable insurance statement program, then you will find yourself scurrying around for the "right" form.

ADEQUATE SUPPLIES

In most systems the printer will get far greater use than that of a typical office typewriter. Volumes of reports may be generated, using up boxes of green bar and ribbons and wearing out Daisy Wheels. Take a look at the end of Chapter 11. There a recommended list of supplies is given. Sufficient quantities will prevent work delays and hurry-up calls or trips to supply houses. Don't worry about having an extra carton of ribbons or green bar. You will use it!

Chapter 6
Backups

A SHORT STORY WITH A LONG LEGACY
HOW TO MAKE EFFICIENT BACKUPS
   Floppy Disk Backups
   Hard Disk Backups
   Long-Range Backups

A SHORT STORY WITH A LONG LEGACY

The heartbreak of psoriasis is nothing compared to the agony of destroying a disk that has not been backed up. A backup is an exact copy of all or part of the information stored on a disk. The following account was given by a remorseful radiologist shortly after accidentally erasing a word processing diskette.

> We've been backing up the MOS as frequently as two to three times a day. But the word processing hadn't been backed up for a week. We had been pressed for time, and it didn't seem as though we were adding that much data. I thought perhaps I'd back up the word processing at the end of that day, but I inadvertently destroyed the diskette shortly before noon. I ended up looking up at a stack of hard copy on green bar that needed to be "retyped" and would take another 8 to 10 hours to do. It included correspondence and complex reports. Each day we had added about 5 or 6 pages of material, and the loss had gradually mounted to about 35 pages.
>
> The error was simple enough. My secretary wanted to start a fresh word processing disk. The problem was that, as the "resident computer specialist and systems analyst," I accidentally reformatted the current disk and wiped out all the data on it. It would have been more convenient if I could have blamed my secretary. In a fit of righteousness I could have told her to be more careful, perhaps take off the rest of the day (to complete my punishment).

The manual's documentation for making backups was vague, and I chose the wrong keystrokes, so, alas, I could only wallow in a certain degree of self-pity as I contemplated the waste of time and money resulting in not backing up the disk prior to the reformatting procedure. Of course, I could rationalize it and say, "Well, if we were working with the old typewriter, it would just be a lot of first drafts that had to be retyped and rechecked anyway." But that was $15,000 ago.

Three things saved this doctor from having a minor disaster become a major one:

1. There was an old backup, true, it was a week old, but matters would have been worse if it had been two weeks old.
2. The doctor had been printing word processing directories regularly, so he could see which data were lost and which were saved.
3. Hard copy rough drafts had been saved and could be used for retyping.

The lesson is: No matter how time consuming it may appear—make backups. Hindsight will always reveal that doing so would have been worth it. Most experts say you will make the mistake of neglecting backups only once.

HOW TO MAKE EFFICIENT BACKUPS

There are two routines that are used for backing up—one for floppy, the other for hard disk. Business application programs are disseminated on floppy disks, so with very few exceptions both floppy and hard disk users will incorporate programs by placing them in the floppy disk drive. Floppy users will continue to operate from the floppy drive; however, hard disk users will transfer information from floppy to hard disk and operate from hard disk thereafter. Both types of disk users will immediately make a backup of the original floppy application programs, remove the write protection tab from the disk (thus prohibiting it from being altered), and store the disk someplace safe for use only under special circumstances.

Floppy Disk Backups

In addition to the above procedures, which both floppy and hard disk users will follow, the subsequent procedures are for floppy users. A triple-rotation backup is recommended. This involves the use of three disks for each application disk that also contains data, all data disks, and all pairings of application and data disks that are altered simultaneously. The three disks are labeled A, B, and C. Let's say you start with a word processing disk, called WPD. That disk would be labeled WPD–A. When you have finished using it, it is backed up onto WPD–B. WPD–A is then stored in a box with all the A backups. However, because you will be using WPD–B next, it is placed in a box labeled "Today." The next time you use word processing, you go to the Today box to get your latest backup, which just happens to be WPD–B. You use it. When you are finished, you back it up onto a disk labeled WPD–C. WPD–B is then tucked away in box B, and WPD–C (which is your latest backup) is placed in the Today box. This system assures that there is always a third disk available that is not involved in the backup routine and cannot be inadvertently ruined should something untoward occur during the backup. The "four box system" A–B–C–Today is an easy method of identifying the latest and oldest disks.

Hard Disk Backups

Recent developments make the backup procedure even easier for hard disk than it is for floppy. Data are backed up to floppy, but in condensed form. Simple instructions also allow you to back up only modified files. Thus, it is not necessary to have multiple saves of identical information. Depending on the volume of data, it is possible to back up a hard disk drive operation with only three to five disks, representing a daily save, a weekly save, and a monthly save. Some hard disks may be backed up to tape cassettes. This procedure is even less complicated than backing up to floppy.

Long-Range Backups

In addition to having the backups indicated above, it is advisable to store monthly and yearly saves for as many years as you would save tax receipts or canceled checks. By now, it should be apparent that a hidden cost to the user is that of the floppy disks themselves. Depending on the volume of data entry and on the degree of the user's dedication, it is possible to have a collection of more than 200 backup diskettes in a few years.

This is one of the shortest chapters but probably the most important in this book. It must always be remembered that no matter how fancy the machine, storage is ultimately being done by a volatile electromagnetic medium. Whether data are lost because of operator error, power failure or surge, or a ringing telephone placed too close, the result without a backup is probably universal—a stew made from lots of scraps of wasted time and money seasoned with an ample quantity of remorse.

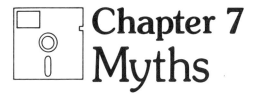

Chapter 7
Myths

THE PURCHASE OF A COMPUTER SYSTEM
   FOLLOWS A SCIENTIFIC STUDY
IT'S EXPENSIVE
IT'S INEXPENSIVE
IT'S COMPLICATED
IT'S SIMPLE
IT SAVES TIME
HARD DISK DRIVE WILL MAKE YOUR COMPUTER
   AS FAST AS A MAINFRAME
TURNKEY OPERATIONS ARE TROUBLE-FREE

For a field that is so precise, a lot of mythology has grown up around computer science. This chapter explores the common myths about the use of microcomputers in private practice.

THE PURCHASE OF A COMPUTER SYSTEM FOLLOWS A SCIENTIFIC STUDY

A psychiatrist relates the following story:

> Before I purchased my first IBM Selectric typewriter and dictating machine in 1970, a representative first came to my office. He met with me and my secretary and proceeded to do a study of our word processing needs. A few days later he produced a report showing how the IBM typewriter and dictating machine would actually reduce the cost of our operation. I then felt justified in making what seemed to be an enormous investment of nearly $1,400 in word processing equipment.
>
> Because I am still using the same IBM typewriter and dictating machine that I did in 1970, it was natural for me to call IBM when I became interested in getting a computer for my office. I was hoping

to get a modern-day version of the salesman who came to my office then. I figured a salesman would be delighted to come by. After all, the equipment was likely to be 5 to 10 times more costly than my original setup.

When I called IBM and they ascertained that I was not going to use a computer to track missiles or set up an automobile-manufacturing firm, they gave me a number in Boca Raton of their personal computer division. I called down there, some 1,500 miles away. A pleasant-sounding fellow gave me another number in a city nearby. It was for Computerland. No one there was interested in coming to my office to do a study about my office needs. However, when I went to Computerland, there was an array of computers and salesmen. I was greeted by neither. Alas, progress!

There are books with charts and systems that purportedly assist the practitioner in determining whether or not he would benefit from computerization, and if so, what size system he would need (see the annotated bibliography). There is a bit of compulsiveness in these schemes that may not be either necessary or beneficial. The formula for decision making need not be complex.

A solo practitioner grossing under $700 a week will probably do just fine with an adding machine, account cards, and a good typewriter. If he files fewer than 50 insurance forms a month, it is debatable whether a computer is going to do the job more efficiently than a secretary. From a cost point of view, it is certainly obvious that for such a small operation an $800 typewriter is going to be more efficient than a $10,000 word processor/microcomputer.

To some degree, measuring the time involved in producing forms and tabulations may be helpful. However, any practice consisting of 1–10 practitioners that generates more than 10 pages of correspondence or reports per week and runs between 100 and 1,000 insurance forms and patient statements combined per month can benefit from a microcomputer system, whose cost ranges between $8,000 and $20,000, including software.

In fact, the computer is likely to be helpful in areas that are difficult to measure at all. Although it is possible to compare the relative time it takes to produce correspondence with a standard typewriter and with a computer, what about the time involved in reviewing patients' accounts to determine their age and status? Most MOS packages can produce a written report giving patient balances and ages of accounts. In addition, the MOS user can request report variations. For example, instead of a complete report, a practitioner can produce one giving only balances of over $100 for more than 60 days. Within a few minutes, it is possible to determine the status of dozens of accounts and to decide what should be done about them. The method is so easy, so efficient, that in order to stimulate continued cash flow many doctors will sit down with their bookkeeper or secretary for two half-hour periods each week with these readouts. Nearly any noncomputerized method involves tedious sorting through account or ledger cards that may have to be manually extricated and refiled. Moreover, if records are kept manually, the aging of the bill (how much of the bill is 30 days old, 60 days old, 90 days old, etc.) may not be readily apparent, especially if the patient is ongoing.

The old methods are so tedious and time consuming that such checks may be made less frequently, and certainly less thoroughly. It is the ability of the computer to perform such tedious tasks at lightning speed that makes it worthwhile. In truth, there may be little point to comparisons between "the old methods" and "the computer method." No amount of compulsive charting will provide specific figures, because the use of computers will inevitably lead to cost-saving procedures that were impossible without them.

IT'S EXPENSIVE

Not long ago, a colleague of mine mentioned that he had bought a computer for his unwieldy multimember pediatric practice. When he told me that the system cost $85,000, my heart sank like a stone. Perhaps his computer does everything, including making breakfast for the staff, but nowadays, systems that cost over $25,000 are usually reserved for hospitals. With advances in technology, most $5,000 computers can now do what a $250,000 computer did 20 years ago—and do it better.

IT'S INEXPENSIVE

Maybe $15,000 is inexpensive to you, and if so, then computers are inexpensive. Certainly, give up thinking about running your practice on a Commodore VIC–64 or an ATARI 800. These "under $1,000 systems" lack the sophistication needed to run a medical office. It is possible to get a computer for under $2,500 if your principal aim is word processing. However, systems that fully integrate the financial, information retrieval, and word processing functions necessary to run a medical office will cost a bare bones minimum of $6,000 and are more likely to cost over $10,000.

IT'S COMPLICATED

One does not have to learn auto mechanics to drive a car well. It is also not necessary to learn computer programming or become a systems analyst in order to use a computer effectively. There are fundamentals that need to be learned, most of them can be studied from manuals or learned by instruction, and the rest can be picked up by experience. Packages are available that meet 99.9 percent of the doctor's software needs. Even if programming modification is needed, it is often more time efficient to get a $25-an-hour consultant than try to do it yourself.

IT'S SIMPLE

Some computer companies would have you believe that it's as easy to run their equipment and software as it is to turn on an oven. It's probably more correct to say that it is as easy to learn to operate an MOS as it is to learn to play chess. (Note that I did not say it was as easy as becoming a master at chess—just to play it.) There are fundamental rules and strategies that must be learned and followed. Errors are simple to make, often difficult to detect, and invariably result in loss of time and information. There is probably no system available that can be learned in less than a month. And in truth, the time is more like three months.

IT SAVES TIME

This may be one of the funniest myths of all—one that veteran computer users and salespersons secretly laugh up their sleeves about. For the first 90 days, the computer will not save you any time at all. It will add on time. Until the computer gets going, you will have to enter transactions into both your old system and the computer system. Because most software programs are not designed to completely replace the commonly used day sheets, entry into both systems may go on indefinitely. Your initial use of the computer system will certainly be more burdensome than time-saving. In addition, there is a tendency to fill up time saved by computerized word processing. Because it is so easy to correct drafts, there is often a trend to produce more correspondence or make more corrections. It's only when you need to collate and reproduce information in the form of insurance bills or patient statements that the computer system will start to show its power and speed.

HARD DISK DRIVE WILL MAKE YOUR COMPUTER AS FAST AS A MAINFRAME

Hard disk drives will make your operations faster (see Chapter 4), but their speed is greatly overrated. The user will be disappointed if she spends $3,000–$4,000 on a hard disk drive expecting to have information appear on the screen as fast as a keystroke. There are, however, advantages to hard disk drives other than speed. These are listed in Chapter 4.

TURNKEY OPERATIONS ARE TROUBLE-FREE

In a turnkey operation the doctor pays a firm to come in and set everything up for her. Supposedly the doctor only needs to know how to turn on the computer. From there on, the operation is trouble-free, or at least made trouble-free by the consultant. The doctor pays a premium for not having to tinker with the system or become very knowledgeable about computer theory and practice.

Although some consulting firms have produced satisfied customers, there are long lists of doctors who have acquired so-called turnkey systems and met with frustration and worse (see Chapter 10). The recent surge in microcomputer manufacturing is relatively new, but the surge in microcomputer consulting is even newer. Stories of blatant fraud are quite rare, but there are abundant accounts of unfulfilled contracts and consultant bankruptcies. Any doctor wishing to acquire a computer system for her office had better resign herself not only to becoming knowledgeable about her computer but to devoting hours to problem solving when problems arise.

On the whole, the myths that we have uncovered here are not devastating. For the most part, computers deliver reliable, rapid service along a narrow continuum. Properly used, computers will increase your efficiency and your cash flow. Just know what to expect!

Chapter 8
A Typical Day with the Computer

A TYPICAL DAY
INTERVIEW WITH MS. HENNESSY, COMPUTER USER
INTERVIEW WITH DR. REED, COMPUTER OWNER

A TYPICAL DAY

In this chapter you will not only learn how a computer is used in the office, but you will also become familiar with typical terms and operations. If you are already a computer user, you may want to skip the chapter.

Ms. Hennessy is Dr. Reed's secretary and has been with Dr. Reed for five years. Dr. Reed is a psychiatrist in a practice that she owns. Two therapists work for her. Among the three of them, they have about 90 individual patient hours a week, plus see 20 patients a week in groups. By most standards, this is considered a good-sized practice.

About eight months ago, Dr. Reed installed a computer in the business office. It was rough going for the first six weeks, but at present both Dr. Reed and Ms. Hennessy feel confident about the computer and its advantages. The following is a typical day.

The first thing Ms. Hennessy will do this morning is remove the dustcovers from the computer and the printer. Dustcovers are one of the most inexpensive and most important features in computer care. Dust, cigarette smoke, and excessive humidity and temperature are all enemies of the computer. Dust causes insidious damage—sometimes not noticed until months later. Both Ms. Hennessy and Dr. Reed have learned to be "compulsive" about using covers.

Next, a "power-up" procedure is followed. The computer is switched on first, then the printer. The first message that will appear on the screen (the CRT) will be, "Insert disk." This message prompts Ms. Hennessy to insert one of perhaps a dozen floppy disks that store information. She uses separate disks for various functions, such as word processing, the general ledger, and the Medical Office System. This morning Ms. Hennessy will be working with the medical office system disk, which she inserts into the disk drive. Every computer has special instructions on the proper way to insert the disk, so care is taken during this procedure. Once the disk has been inserted, the disk drive "boots" it, which involves verifying whether it is compatible or usable in this computer system. (For example, an IBM computer will reject a Radio Shack disk, and vice versa.) Then Ms. Hennessy is prompted to enter the date and time. The system is now "ready," and she is told so on the video display terminal (VDT or CRT). She types in a short code that brings the MOS program forward, displaying the first menu on the CRT.

Menus are a system of prompts. A menu may be found along the bottom of the screen of each page displayed, or it may take up the center portion of the screen and be displayed independently. The following is the menu Ms. Hennessy sees:

      MAIN MENU

      1 - DAILY INPUT
      2 - DAILY RECAP
      3 - INSURANCE FORMS
      4 - PATIENT STATEMENTS
      5 - A/R REPORT
      6 - ACTIVITY OVERVIEW
      7 - REPORTS MENU
      8 - PATIENT RECALL
      9 - MAINTENANCE MENU
      X - EXIT
         ENTER SELECTION

A menu permits rapid movement within the program, usually by a single keystroke. Sometimes a choice at one menu will lead to a submenu. For example, choice 7, "Reports menu," on the above menu brings up a submenu with the following choices:

```
         REPORTS MENU
         1 - DIAGNOSIS FILE
         2 - PROCEDURE FILE
         3 - PATIENT FILE
         4 - ACCOUNT SUMMARY
         5 - MAILING LABELS
         6 - TRANSACTION REVIEW
         U - MAIN MENU
         X - EXIT
```

This morning Ms. Hennessy will use the MOS four ways. She will (1) enter information on two new patients, (2) enter yesterday's financial transactions, (3) print a report of current accounts receivable, and (4) print insurance forms to be sent out later in the day.

To enter information about the new patients, she presses choice 1, "Daily input." There are a few prompts or questions from the computer. Once the prompts have been answered, the secretary finds an empty "electronic filing card" and enters information about the patient in the same way that she would on any preprinted form. In this program she is prompted to insert the patient's name, address, insurance company, marital status, and other information that might be used in billing or in managing the patient file (see Figure 8–1).

This task completed, Ms. Hennessy enters financial transactions from the previous day. Notice in the illustration that there are prompts along the bottom of the screen. It will not be necessary for Ms. Hennessy to go back to the main menu to enter transactions. All she does is find the file of the patient for whom she wishes to enter transactions. This is done with a few simple keystrokes. Each file will have the same prompts at the bottom of the page. Today Ms. Hennessy will record a $50 charge for Mr. Max O'Herrin. She will bring Mr. O'Herrin's file forward to the screen and press T for transaction (see Figure 8–2). Mr. O'Herrin's

FIGURE 8–1
Patient Record*

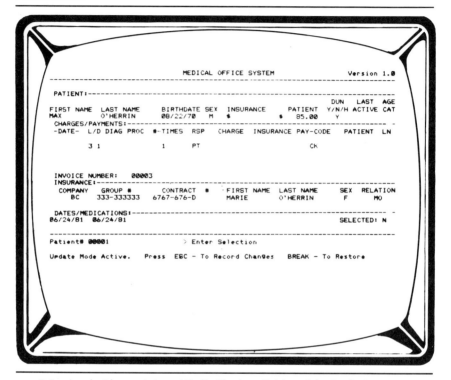

* Reprinted with permission of Radio Shack, a division of the Tandy Corporation.

account card then comes forward, and she enters the appropriate information. This procedure is followed for each patient whose file requires entries.

You may be wondering why the secretary did not enter this information at the time the patient made the payment. This may come as a disappointment to some, but usually a computer system will not replace manual entry onto day sheets. Unless a terminal is dedicated to such data entry and is staffed by someone who is primarily involved in keeping the books, it is impractical to enter information in segments as patients come and go from the office. This is especially true for floppy disk operations (see Chapter 4 for explanation of the difference between floppy and hard disk). It may be convenient to do this if the MOS happens to be up and running on the computer and the menu choice is for "Patient transactions." But let's say the secretary has been using the com-

FIGURE 8-2
Transaction Record*

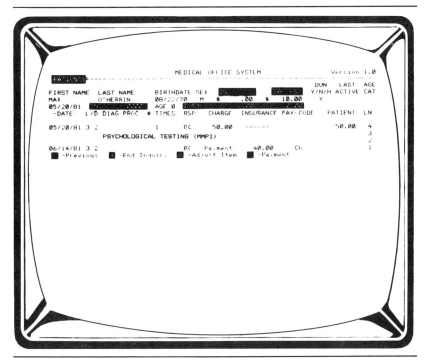

* Reprinted with permission of Radio Shack, a division of the Tandy Corporation.

puter for general ledger and it is going through a half-hour posting period. For a single-user system, there would be no way to access the MOS program until the computer finishes posting general ledger. Even if the computer were finished with the posting, it would still take several minutes to remove the general ledger diskette, insert and boot the MOS diskette, go to the right menu item, unload the MOS diskette, and reload the general ledger diskette and continue working on it.

Before Ms. Hennessy presses option 5 at the main menu for an accounts receivable report, she loads 132-column-wide green bar paper into the printer. This paper is about 14 inches wide and is used for financial reporting. Green bar refers to the green stripe that is printed horizontally across computer paper to assist in reading figures after they are printed. Once the paper has been loaded and option 5 pressed at the main menu, the accounts receivable program is brought forward. By answering a few prompts, Ms. Hennessy instructs the computer to list details on all accounts that are older than 60 days. The printing occurs almost immediately, listing patients' names, account numbers, and transactions, followed by the amounts and ages of balances. Addresses and telephone numbers may also be printed on this page. (See Appendix B for example of A/R report.) Usually a hundred patient accounts can be printed in a few minutes. When the report is finished, the computer automatically displays the main menu on the screen.

Next, Ms. Hennessy will print insurance forms. (See Appendix B for example of Health Insurance Claim Form.) Before she presses option 3 to go to insurance form printing, she loads AMA Form HCFA 1500/CHAMPUS 501 (C-3) into the printer. These are continuous-run "pin" forms. The pinholes are on either side of the form and are grabbed by the "tractor" of the printer. This device assures that the paper is properly aligned in the printer even after a hundred runs. Now Ms. Hennessy presses option 3 to bring up the insurance program. By answering a series of simple prompts, she indicates that she wishes to print all patients, A–Z, whose forms will be submitted to Blue Shield. The first form produced will be a dummy with Xs printed in certain places to ascertain proper alignment. A single key is then pressed. Depending on the number of forms to be printed and the speed of the printer, the system may then run independently, filling in forms for the next 15 minutes to two hours.

Today's run takes a half hour. In this time, the secretary reviews the accounts receivable report with Dr. Reed. Decisions are made regarding the disposition of these accounts.

For now, Ms. Hennessy is finished working with the MOS. Time has passed quickly, and it is already 11 o'clock. She is amazed at how quickly time passes when she is working with the computer. Ms. Hennessy swears she is going to get a little clock to put next to the computer so she can "stay in touch with reality." The tendency is not to take a break. She does not feel she has been working that long, and she is anxious to get on to the next item of business—word processing. She would like to correct a few letters before lunch.

Before taking out the MOS diskette, she "exits" properly by pressing the right keys (by menu prompts) to close all the files and to "bring it all the way back" until the CRT displays DOS-Ready

(Disk Operating System—Ready). Before she removes the MOS diskette, she places another diskette marked "MOS/Backup B" in the second drive. She then enters the command to make a copy of the MOS diskette in the first drive on the backup diskette now in the second drive. This process will take about 15 minutes, which she uses to call the patients whom she reviewed with the doctor during her briefing about accounts receivable. She will ask them about payment. After making a few calls, she glances at the CRT and notices that the words "Backup completed" are displayed. She removes the diskette from the second drive, labels it, puts it carefully into a sleeve, and places the sleeve in a box marked "Today." The next time she uses the MOS she will use the MOS/Backup B diskette that she just put in the Today box. She also removes the MOS diskette in the first drive. With a felt tip pen she carefully labels this diskette as MOS/Backup A. It will be stored in a box where all Backup A's are kept. She uses a felt tip pen so as not to damage the delicate diskette. Now she is ready to do some word processing.

She removes her word processing diskette from the Today box and places it in the first disk drive. At "DOS-Ready" she types I- ENTER to initialize this diskette. It is not necessary for her to start from scratch. Initialization takes about 10 seconds, and this diskette now becomes electronically marked with the same date as the MOS diskette.

Dr. Reed has given Ms. Hennessy five pages of green bar consisting of two letters and a three-page report; all of the pages have some corrections. Following menu prompts, Ms. Hennessy "finds" these letters and the report on the diskette. With a few keystrokes she is able to make the required corrections, which include adding and deleting characters and words and moving sentences around. To make sure that everything is correct, she places a spelling dictionary diskette in the second drive. She presses a key to activate the program, which will check the spelling of the work she has just finished.

When Ms. Hennessy is certain that the correspondence is in order, she places a sheet of letterhead in the printer and aligns it. With a few keystrokes on the computer, the first letter is printed—letter-perfect—in 26 seconds. A similar process is followed for the second and third letters. For the report the printer pauses at the end of each page, waiting for the secretary to reload a sheet of white bond paper and "press Y to continue." Ms. Hennessy glances at the clock and is amazed to find that it is already 12:25 P.M. She removes the spelling dictionary from the second drive and returns it to the Today box. She places a word processing diskette marked "Word Processing B" in the second drive. At DOS-Ready Ms. Hennessy types a one-line command instructing the computer to back up the first drive onto the second drive. This a good time to take lunch. The computer does not need attending while the backup procedure is going on. When Ms. Hennessy returns at 1:30 P.M., she glances at the CRT. It reads, "Backup complete."

Now Ms. Hennessy will be doing some transcription. The diskette in the first disk drive, marked "Word Processing A," is put in a box with the other A backups. Ms. Hennessy takes Word Processing B (the latest backup) out of the second disk drive and places it in the first disk drive. If something bad should happen to Word Processing B, she will be able to go to the box marked "A Backups" and pull out Word Processing A. Once again, the diskette just placed in the first drive is initialized by pressing I- (ENTER) at the main menu. Ms. Hennessy follows the prompts to create a "new document." In this procedure she finds that "typing" is similar to ordinary typing but that it goes faster because it is easier to correct mistakes and because there is no need to hit a carriage return.

Interspersed with the letters and reports are case notes, but it has been decided to use a standard typewriter for case notes. Before Dr. Reed became a computer user, she had dreamed about "putting all the records on the computer." In fact, when she got the computer, she attempted this. But since she was using floppy disks and a single terminal, Dr. Reed soon ran into problems. In the first place, the case notes soon filled up several floppy diskettes and indexing them became cumbersome. Second, when she wanted to look at case notes, it was necessary to disrupt the secretary, who might then be using the computer for something else. Third, it was already necessary to maintain hard copy files of incoming correspondence and forms for patients. The old method of going to the patient's chart, taking the last sheet of notes, placing it in the typewriter, and adding new notes on to it took no longer than using the word processing program. Besides, note corrections did not have to be as neat as corrections of copy that was being sent out of the office. Ms. Hennessy also found that it was just as easy to type envelopes in the conventional way if only two or three needed to be done. However, mass envelope typing was reserved for the computer and printer. And, in fact, later in the day she would print 100 labels in about 45 seconds.

It is already 2:15 P.M., and there is lots more work to be done. The day sheets have to be balanced. Dr. Reed had spent several mornings developing an electronic spread sheet that would help the secretary balance the day sheets. Ms. Hennessy loads this program and with a couple of keystrokes brings forward a blank spread sheet especially designed by the doctor. The figures are quickly transferred from the day sheet to the electronic spread sheet. As the figures are entered, they are automatically tabulated and proven. Any errors are immediately flagged by the computer for the secretary's attention. This task used to take about 20 minutes per page, and sometimes much longer if there were errors that could not be detected. This afternoon Ms. Hennessy completes three pages in 20 minutes, including the electronic transfer of the data onto a master spread sheet that enables Dr. Reed to examine the cash flow status of the practice from week to week and month to month.

After finishing this task, Ms. Hennessy goes through the same backup routine with this program as she did with word processing and MOS earlier in the day. While the computer is doing the backup, she files correspondence and reports.

It is now 3:00 P.M. In the remaining two hours Ms. Hennessy will utilize the computer to (1) send personally typed letters to 20 past-due accounts, providing specific information in each letter about the status of the account; (2) print 100 address labels; and (3) create a form letter to be duplicated for 100 CHAMPUS and Blue Cross patients. She removes the electronic spread sheet diskette and backup from the computer. She reloads the word processing program and corrects the final draft of a letter that will explain changes in the billing procedure to all CHAMPUS and Blue Cross patients. It is produced letter-perfect in the printer and will then be taken to the Xerox machine for duplication.

Before Ms. Hennessy does this, she unloads the word processing program. She has decided that not enough information has been entered on the word processing diskette to warrant waiting 20 minutes for a backup. She reloads the MOS, however, and brings up the label addressing program. She loads address labels into the printer, and after alignment she presses a few keys telling the computer to print address labels for all active CHAMPUS and Blue Cross patients. As the printer starts the labels, she sets the Xerox machine for 100 copies so that the form letter and labels will be finished at about the same time. A few minutes later she takes the labels from the printer and puts them with the finished form letters. She will stuff the envelopes and affix labels in a little while.

While the MOS is in the first disk drive, she places the word processing diskette in the second drive. On the word processing diskette she already has a "merge letter" that leaves room for patient names and addresses and a place to provide information about how much the patient owes and how many days overdue the account is. She now loads Dr. Reed's letterhead onto the printer. This time she is using continuous-run paper, perforated so that, when "burst," it will be indiscernible from regular paper. With a few more keystrokes the computer is instructed to type letters to all patients having a balance of more than $50 for more than 45 days but not more than 60 days. Older accounts will get a different letter. One after another, the printer types these letters, each of which takes about 25 seconds. While Ms. Hennessy is keeping an eye on the printer to make sure that there are no difficulties (such as the printing ribbon running out or the paper jamming), she folds the form letters run off by the Xerox machine, stuffs them in the envelopes, and affixes labels and stamps.

It is now about 4:40 P.M. Ms. Hennessy unloads all the programs, powers down the computer, places dustcovers over the printer and the computer, and informs the answering service that the office is closing for the day. She gathers the mail, which consists of several packets to go to insurance companies, a bundle of form letters to go to CHAMPUS and Blue Cross patients, and a stack of 20 letters to go to a group of past-due accounts.

In this example, Ms. Hennessy did not have to answer telephone calls or interact with patients. In most one- or two-secretary offices, the procedures described above will be interrupted by other activities. The example, however, does demonstrate two things. First, the computer can speed up mechanical and tedious procedures. Second, computers do have limitations. A $10,000 floppy disk single-user computer operation is not going to permit all staff members to do all things at all times. A multi-user system gives much more versatility, but it also costs much more. Multi-user systems are explained in Chapter 15.

INTERVIEW WITH MS. HENNESSY, COMPUTER USER

Let's take a moment to interview Ms. Hennessy and Dr. Reed and get their reactions to the above computer system.

INTERVIEWER: What was your reaction when Dr. Reed told you she was thinking about getting a computer?
MS. HENNESSY: Dr. Reed had been thinking about it for a long time and had been doing lots of reading on it. In fact, she had given me some articles to read myself. She never told me she was getting a computer. Rather, she asked me what I thought about getting one.
INTERVIEWER: And your reaction?
HENNESSY: I thought it was a good idea. In fact, I was a little excited about it. Two of my friends had been working with word processors for a year or so, and they liked it. I saw this as a way of growing professionally. You hear so much about computers; I thought it was time I learned about them myself.
INTERVIEWER: Besides doing some reading, how else did you prepare for using the computer.
HENNESSY: Actually, I did quite a bit of reading. Most of the things I read were supplied by Dr. Reed. The ones I found most helpful were popular books on the topic that were not too technical. A few weeks before the computer arrived, Dr. Reed and I and one other staff person took a series of courses. There was a brief course on how to run the computer, and there were a few other courses. The most important one, however, was a two-day course on word processing.
INTERVIEWER: Did you have any fears?
HENNESSY: Yes, I had the usual ones, I suppose. First, I had some doubts as to whether I could learn to use the computer. I had been with Dr. Reed for over five years and pretty much run the office myself; the typewriter had become an extension of my fingers. I didn't look forward to the prospect of changing everything around and maybe not being able to do a good job. But I have somewhat of an adventuresome nature, so I was able to overcome that fear. The other fear had to do with worrying about the computer taking over. With computers being so fast, I felt that it might make my hours shorter.
INTERVIEWER: Did your hours become shorter?

HENNESSY: Not at all. In fact, during the first month I put in about six hours overtime each week. We had to run our old system and the new system side by side for a while, so some things required almost twice as much work.

INTERVIEWER: Did your fear about making mistakes materialize?

HENNESSY: Yes [*she smiles*]. What Dr. Reed and I both learned is that we made plenty of mistakes. What made things much easier for me was when Dr. Reed accidentally destroyed the data from one of our floppy disks while trying to make a backup. It was a small disaster that took about 10 hours to make right again. But it really cleared the air. After that, I was less concerned about what *I* might do.

INTERVIEWER: What advantages do you see in being a computer user?

HENNESSY: I'm better able to organize the office. The quality of our correspondence has improved considerably. With our electronic proof-reading program, I don't believe any letters or reports have gone out of this office with a typographical error. Our accounts receivable situation is under much better control. We are able to get up-to-the-minute status reports about accounts receivable, not just a global total, but as much detail as we want, including the ages of the various invoices. It makes my work simpler and more efficient, and I know that Dr. Reed is very pleased with the results.

INTERVIEWER: Are there any disadvantages?

HENNESSY: We are still learning about the computer, and from time to time we run into problems and make mistakes that we have to live with.

INTERVIEWER: What are the worst mistakes that occur?

HENNESSY: First of all, nearly any mistake can be undone if you have backup copies of your programs and data that you're storing. But it's not always convenient or efficient to be making backups several times a day. We usually make our backups before lunch or at the end of the day. We have one procedure that's called a monthly purge. It simultaneously rids our system of old paid-up invoices and transfers financial information about the practice into a monthly report format. We are still not certain how we made the error; somehow all of the February and March figures got placed into February. When we look at the reports for the year, March is blank and February is about double. Unfortunately, we did not make a backup prior to this procedure and were stuck with the results.

INTERVIEWER: You were talking about the disadvantages in general.

HENNESSY: There are two other disadvantages that are not major, but they came as a surprise. In the first place, I learned that it's not possible to turn on the computer and use it for a minute or two. There is something about it that is very captivating and makes you forget about time. The other disadvantage is that in some respects Dr. Reed has become more demanding. It is so easy to produce financial reports and redo correspon-

dence that there is a tendency to redo these things more often than we used to.
INTERVIEWER: On the whole, are things better or worse than they were before you became a computer user?
HENNESSY: It's funny, we've only been using the computer about eight months, and it's hard to remember what it was like before. The typewriter rarely gets used; Dr. Reed is developing a program to quickly type envelopes, which except for case notes is one of the few things that you use a typewriter for. Sometimes I miss the old way. It wasn't as efficient, but it was comfortable, like an old shoe. But there's no doubt that the computer is more efficient, and it has improved many aspects of Dr. Reed's practice.

INTERVIEW WITH DR. REED, COMPUTER OWNER

INTERVIEWER: Why did you get a computer for your practice?
DR. REED: I've always had a fascination with electronics; not that I've ever dealt in it, but I've enjoyed reading about it. When the price of computers started to fall two years ago, I began exploring the possibility of using one in the office. At that time, I had very little notion about how I would use it. I had heard about word processing programs and data base management; so I thought there would be some way of using these modern devices in the office.
INTERVIEWER: Did you hesitate at all in purchasing a computer system?
DR. REED: Yes. In fact, I thought about it for a year. During that time, I read as much as I could on the topic and also spoke to people who were either contemplating getting a computer or had one. I really had two concerns after I finally decided to get one. The first was that even though the price was coming down, they were not cheap; and the second was that the prices were continuing to fall with new developments always coming out. I was afraid to get stuck with something that would be too expensive and out-of-date.
INTERVIEWER: At what point did you finally decide to go ahead and buy a computer?
DR. REED: I've had a Sony Betamax for four years. I purchased it for $1,400. It was loaded with many features. Now I could purchase an equivalent machine with even more features for about $900. However, I realized two things. In the first place, I had four years of use and enjoyment out of it. Though I could've waited around for the price to drop, it was definitely an advantage to have the machine and be able to use it when I wanted to. The second thing is that you don't use most of the special features anyway. For example, the Betamax has a 14-day timer on which you can record up to four programs. In point of fact, if

I want to record something, I usually set it in the morning or evening before I go out and record a program that comes on that day. Since that experience, I decided that the same concepts probably apply to computers. Although the price may come down, at least I would have the advantage of using it; and as long as it had features that I wanted, I was not going to become concerned about some special features that future computers might have.

INTERVIEWER: Did you make the right decision to buy a computer when you did?

DR. REED: I'm convinced that I did. In our first month of use the computer "found" nearly $4,000 of "lost" accounts. After four months' use, our accounts receivable picture had been reduced by about 15 percent. The computer has nearly paid for itself in the eight months that we've had it. Waiting around to save a few thousand bucks wouldn't have been as economical as it would've appeared at first. There have been software developments and improvements since we started the system. However, the updated versions have been provided to us without additional cost by the software firm that we're dealing with. Our computer was also bought from a large company that has a reputation for supporting all of its older models and permitting updating of them at a reasonable cost.

INTERVIEWER: Would you do anything differently if you were to start up again?

DR. REED: That's difficult to say. I would certainly go into it with different expectations. Computer use represented a major change in the business aspect of my practice. To some degree, every one of our routines was altered, as was work distribution. Although we adjusted, neither I or my staff was fully prepared for the changes.

INTERVIEWER: Any advice to potential users?

DR. REED: Yes! Hardware and software are easy to shop for, but "support" is not. I went into this thing by myself, buying hardware and software off the shelf, so to speak. I had no idea how long it would take to learn to use the programs. And I had no idea of the number of problems we could run into. Considering that I put in about 10 to 15 extra hours a week for six months to learn our system and make it work well, I've thought that hiring a consultant might have been more efficient. "Next time" I would consider a turnkey operation or at least more formal support.

INTERVIEWER: You have regrets?

DR. REED: Not really. It's fun to complain. In the final analysis, my accounts receivable picture has improved dramatically and my word processing has been turned into a fine art. My practice has never run so smoothly. I feel that I'm light-years ahead of colleagues who are still thinking about getting a computer.

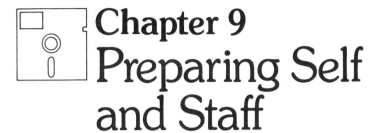

Chapter 9
Preparing Self and Staff

PREPARATION
    Should You Learn How to Program?
    Minimize Changes
PRIOR INVOLVEMENT OF STAFF
    Discussion
    What Training Is Needed?
SEQUENCE OF ORDERING
    Insurance Forms
    Invoice Forms
    Other Supplies
PHYSICAL CONSIDERATIONS
    Electrical Demands
    Furniture Configuration
    Lighting
HANG LOOSE

PREPARATION

Whether you set up your own computer system or have it done by consultants, there is one critical area that is best accomplished by your own efforts: preparation of yourself and your staff for the change.

Besides reading, what should you do to prepare for the new computer? First, you must realize that there is a limit to what you can do prior to having continued hands-on experience with the computer. It's like reading about a vacation spot before you go there. Some of the reading will prepare you for the exigencies. However, the experiences you have while vacationing will be very different from the experience of reading about the vacation spot beforehand. So it is with computer use.

Should You Learn How to Program?

It is not necessary to learn programming, or even BASIC, prior to becoming a computer user. However, it is helpful to understand certain concepts about computer operations. And there is a fundamental vocabulary that is helpful in communicating with other computer users and experts. Some of the more salient concepts and terms are discussed in Chapters 2, 4, and 8 and in the glossary.

Minimize Changes

The most important thing to realize is that the computer will present change—in some respects, dramatic change. It is a fairly well accepted psychological tenet that change—whether it be positive or negative—will result in stress and that there is greater stress when several changes occur at one time. The introduction of a computer is not only likely to affect your daily work routine; it may also be accompanied by the use of new furniture, different printed forms, a change in keyboard feel, reorientation from looking at hard copy on a desk to looking at a vertical cathode ray tube, and so on. To minimize the stress that results from the introduction of a computer, it would be helpful to postpone nonrelated changes. Introducing a computer at the same time that you are moving to a new office or taking on a new partner would be begging for trouble.

PRIOR INVOLVEMENT OF STAFF

Discussion

Involving staff in the acquisition of a computer is helpful. If the computer is presented as a fait accompli, there may be resistance to it. Employees will have feelings and concerns about the computer. There should be an ongoing forum to discuss these matters. The point is that most members of your staff know that the potential of the computer goes beyond the piece of machinery itself. They sense that a computer can perform many tasks, though they may not yet have the savvy to refer to this as "multiple-programs execution." There may be fears of an inability to perform well with the computer or fears that the computer will take over or lessen their roles. It may be less important to dissuade staff from such concerns than to give staff an opportunity to express them.

What Training Is Needed?

Some formal training will be necessary for anyone who is going to operate a computer. This training may be obtained on site from a consultant, or it may be obtained by attending classes elsewhere. Two of the most common courses on computers are the ones that involve operation of the computer and use of a word processing program. The necessary training should be an integral part of the employee's job. In other words, employees should be paid while they receive the training and should not be expected to do this on their own time. Such a policy will reduce the resentment that may accompany the change to a computer system.

SEQUENCE OF ORDERING

Even if your system is set up by a consulting firm, certain items may not be on hand when the computer is finally up and running. These are listed below.

Insurance Forms

The computer will print out on insurance forms especially designed for continuous feeding into the print tractor. If you do not have a user-modifiable insurance form program, it may be necessary to acquire a specific form. (This could take up to six weeks.) Almost all programs utilize form HCFA 1500/CHAMPUS 501 (C–3), see Appendix B, which is usually available from most large insurance carriers (e.g., Blue Cross/Blue Shield) or the American Medical Association. But securing these forms will still take time. It will also be necessary to make special arrangement with insurance carriers so that you may print "Signature on file" in the place marked for the patient's signature instead of having the patient sign each form. This procedure may take as long as a month to set up, and it usually requires having patients sign special forms and keeping the forms on file.

Invoice Forms

Continuous-run invoice forms can be bought "off the shelf" and do not have to be personally imprinted. However, such forms will probably be available off the shelf only in large cities and your supplier may have to order them for you.

Other Supplies

At the end of Chapter 11 there is a list of commonly used supplies. It is worth checking. Two items that new computer systems often lack are diskettes for backups and continuous-run labels.

PHYSICAL CONSIDERATIONS

Electrical Demands

It's a good idea (but not essential) to have a separate, or "dedicated," line to the computer system. Power surges may damage the computer; power loss invariably results in data loss. A vacuum cleaner, refrigerator, or air conditioner may do either of these things. Having the computer electrically separated from these appliances will reduce the potential for problems.

Furniture Configuration

Existing furniture and its placement usually do not work well for computers. The furniture may not be sturdy enough, especially for a Daisy Wheel printer. Because of the vibration caused by printers, printers and computers do not belong on the same table. Many printers cannot be placed against a wall, as they need front *and* back access for paper loading and accumulation. Computer operations abound with cables, which present both an aesthetic and a safety problem. It is important that the furniture used in computer operations be specially designed and carefully placed.

Lighting

Most modern offices have the wrong type of lighting for computer use.[1] Their light walls, bright fluorescent lights, and white furniture

---

[1] Joel Makover, "Terminal Illnesses," in *Office Hazards* (Washington, D.C.: Tilden Press, 1981) pp.85–108.

increase eyestrain for the CRT user. When a secretary must look back and forth from brightly lit paper copy to a relatively dim CRT, the rapid changes in the opening of the iris result in eyestrain and fatigue. It is generally recommended that office lighting around the CRT be indirect and about half the intensity of the lighting in a "normal" office. Incandescent flood lights directed away from the CRT and connected to dimmers are preferable to fluorescent lights. Intense natural lighting (windows) can be a problem too. The trick is to reduce glare from the CRT while producing enough lighting to see the work.

In the absence of ideal lighting, an antiglare screen add-on may be helpful. This will reduce glare. Also helpful are CRTs whose positions can be changed, detachable keyboards, and movable easels to hold work.

HANG LOOSE

And finally, it's helpful to have a *que sera sera* attitude. Being patient with yourself and your staff will go a long way toward easing the transition to the computer. Although exciting and useful, that transition will bring many opportunities to test your frustration level and that of your staff.

In the next two chapters you will learn exactly how to go about setting up the system.

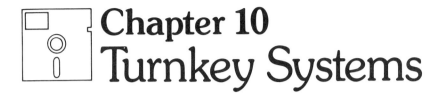

Chapter 10
Turnkey Systems

A MATTER OF FINANCES
GUIDELINES
   Custom-Made
      Software
      Hardware
   Support
   Costs
   Time
   Proximity
   Financial Stability
   Labeling Oranges and Apples

A MATTER OF FINANCES

Dr. Fitzpatrick was interested but cautious. She realized the potential of a computer for her practice, but she also realized her own limitations. She was a busy professional, and her time would be better spent in managing and developing her clinical practice than in learning how to program and run a computer system. The commonsense approach for her was to hire a computer consulting firm to install a system and get it running. But Dr. Fitzpatrick was aware of the dangers of this approach. A medical treatment center for which she sometimes provided services had had a terrible experience with a consulting firm. This small firm was engaged to install a "tailor-made" system. Not long after the equipment was delivered, the company went out of business. The treatment center was stuck with a 16-bit central processing unit, two terminals, a printer, modem, some partially completed software, and a $50,000 debit.

85

Dr. Fitzpatrick researched the matter and found a highly reliable consulting firm about 1,000 miles away with about 300 active customers. The firm agreed to provide her with everything she needed, from equipment to instruction. It also offered another attractive feature. If Dr. Fitzpatrick ran into any difficulty with any program, all she would have to do was call up the consulting firm and connect her computer to the consulting firm's computer with the use of a modem; the firm would then correct the difficulty long-distance.

It seemed like a good deal, so Dr. Fitzpatrick signed up. Things didn't go as smoothly as planned, but after arriving piecemeal, the equipment was finally installed. During the first day of instruction, Dr. Fitzpatrick and her staff learned how to enter patient information.

"At least, it's working all right, after all that aggravation!" Dr. Fitzpatrick was heard to say to her secretary at the end of the day.

In her excitement Dr. Fitzpatrick returned to the office early the next day to take a look at the electronic patient records. To her amazement, there were peculiar graphic marks in some of the places where data had been entered. Instead of addresses and telephone numbers, there were things that looked like rows of upside down Rs. At 9 A.M. Dr. Fitzpatrick called the consulting firm, a thousand miles away, and was told, "Don't worry about it; we'll get it fixed." She was then instructed to connect the computer by telephone. "We'll give you a call back when it's all finished."

With some trepidation Dr. Fitzpatrick wished her secretary good luck and left for rounds at the hospital. Upon her return the secretary told her that the consulting firm had called back at about 11 to say that everything was fine. And, in fact, everything did seem to work fine, until three weeks later, when Dr. Fitzpatrick received a letter from the federal Bankruptcy Court indicating that World Wide Computer Consultants had filed for bankruptcy. After a few panic calls, she learned that although the firm had provided fine products and services, it had handled its money unwisely and overinvested in real estate. Fortunately for Dr. Fitzpatrick, her system was operational. Also, when World Wide Computer folded, it was taken over by another firm that honored its contracts. Dr. Fitzpatrick had had a close call.

Although the above stories are true, they are not presented to say, "Don't ever use a consulting firm." They are presented to shed some light on the topic. Buying a computer system to manage your office is *like* driving across the desert. Someone may guarantee that you'll always have your car running, but if the car stops in the middle of the desert and the guarantor is not around, you'd better have the know-how to either get out of that tight spot or to survive while you are waiting for help.

GUIDELINES

It is helpful to use a consulting firm to assist in setting up a system, but there are a number of guidelines and cautions that should be observed. These are discussed below.

Custom-Made

Software. Many consulting firms will provide custom-made software. This service permits idiosyncratic aspects of the practice to be dealt with by the program. A specially designed MOS might cost 10 to 20 times as much as an existing package. For most practices, however, existing software may be utilized without the need for special development. Also, a considerable amount of money may be saved if existing packages are modified, either by the user or a consultant.

The more customized software is, the more dependent the practitioner will become on the consultant. This may not be a problem so long as the consultant is available and the practitioner has the funds to pay for continuing support. However, being able to use existing software, even if provided by a consultant, will give you the advantage of being able to rely on either the consultant or the original software producer.

Hardware. The same cautions regarding custom-made software apply to custom-made hardware. There is so much available in terms of tested computer hardware that the practitioner has little need for custom-made equipment. Specific input devices are a possible exception. For example, it might be convenient to use a special keyboard when administering a psychological test by computer. The keyboard might consist only of large keys marked "True/False," "Yes/No," etc. Even so, most practitioners will find that the special equipment they need is already manufactured.

Support

Support refers to the degree to which a software or hardware manufacturer will help you learn a system, debug it of problems, and come to your aid when you get stuck. Despite what manufacturers would have us believe, computers and computer programs are both complicated and touchy. One must decide on and be able to determine how much support will be needed or expected. Obtaining support is one of the principle reasons for hiring a consulting firm or an individual consultant.

Support can be broken down into two distinct types: initial support and continued support. Initial support involves setting up the equipment, providing basic training in its operation, and providing assistance during the first few days of operation. Continued support involves these services as well as an arrangement under which the consultant will help the user on a continued basis for a specified period of time. Most consulting firms will provide the former, but a practitioner may expect and need the latter.

The following types of support should be expected: (1) preliminary training and office organization and preparation for the installation of the computer system; (2) complete installation of the system, including the testing of all programs; (3) training and instruction in the operation of the equipment and the programs; and (4) periodic on-site consultation to assist with problems as they emerge during the postinstallation period.

Costs

Any practitioner who intends to have a computer system installed but does not intend to become involved in its operation may as well resign himself to spending 100 percent above equipment costs for consultation fees and support.

Time

It is recommended that 24–30 postinstallation hours of on-site consultation be available for use at the rate of four–six hours per week during the first five weeks of operation. After this period, support will be needed only to cope with latent software or hardware problems. A block of four–six hours of consultation might also be scheduled whenever a new program is instituted.

Proximity

Regardless of the sales pitch given, a company that is closer will be able to provide more efficient, less expensive service than a company farther away. A consultant who must fly 1,000 miles each time she provides you with a half day's service will have to be more costly than a consultant in town.

Financial Stability

The more software and equipment a company custom-designs for your office, the more relevant is the financial stability of the company. You will be paying a greater premium not only for the development of these items but also for the consultation necessary for support. You take the risk of having an unusable system if the company goes out of business. A customer list made available to you by the company and an investigation by your accountant of the company's probable stability will help you in determining how great that risk is. The risk becomes proportionally less when (1) equipment and software are provided off the shelf and are developed by well-known companies; (2) you receive direct title of all equipment; and (3) payments to the consultant do not substantially exceed the rate of delivery of materials and services.

Labeling Oranges and Apples

As a hedge against misunderstanding, a written agreement with the consulting firm should differentiate between goods and services. Such labeling will provide a better framework for determining when you are to pay what. You may then pay for services and goods when they are actually delivered. The agreement will go a long way toward protecting the interests of both parties.

Chapter 11
Your Own Turnkey Operation for under $12,500

DO IT YOURSELF
    Radio Shack
    The Catalog
    Seven Fundamental Requirements
    Close to Home
INSTRUCTION
    Operator's Course
    Word Processing Course
    Data Base Course
EQUIPMENT
    Computer
    Keyboard
    Floppy Disk Drives
    Operating System
    Hard Disk Drive
    Printer
    Bidirectional Tractors
    Modem
FURNITURE
SOFTWARE
    Medical Office System
        User Modification
        Document Capacity
        Standard Forms
        User Friendly

Data Bases
Financial Reports
Scripsit
Scripsit Spelling and Hyphenation Dictionary
Profile Plus
Visi-Calc
SUPPLIES
AVOIDING DOWNTIME
Service
Service Contracts
Maintenance
Support
When Things Go Haywire
THE SHOPPING LIST

DO IT YOURSELF

In Chapter 10 turnkey operations were discussed. For a specific price a company provides you with just about everything you need, from hardware to instruction. There is an alternative— creating a "do-it-yourself turnkey operation." Ordinarily, that would be a contradiction in terms, because in a turnkey operation almost everything is done for you initially. This chapter will serve two functions: (1) It will describe in detail every product and service you will need to become a full-fledged computer user. (2) It will provide the prices and catalog numbers of these items and tell you where to get them in one step.

Radio Shack

Radio Shack is in the unique position of offering all kinds of computerware within a few miles of any populated area in the United States. What reader of this book doesn't know where the local Radio Shack is? Most Radio Shack stores have a computer department. But there are also full-fledged Radio Shack "computer stores," dealing solely in microprocessing. At these stores it is possible to get everything you need to run a medical or psychological practice. (Sorry, dentists, they don't carry a dental software package yet, but they carry everything else you need.)

The Catalog

In our household we use the Sears catalog as a reference book. It provides descriptions and pictures of products along with a price that is representative of the products' average price elsewhere. The Radio Shack computer catalog can serve the same function. Whether or not you buy the specific Radio Shack product, the catalog will give you some sense of what it does, how it looks, and what it's likely to cost. In the last section of this chapter Radio Shack catalog numbers and prices are given for each of the items discussed below.

Seven Fundamental Requirements

There are seven fundamental requirements for setting up a computerized office system: instruction, equipment, software, supplies, support, accessories, and service/maintenance. All of these requirements can be met at Radio Shack computer centers and at many regular Radio Shack stores that have a computer department. They can also be met at other stores or combinations of stores in and around large metropolitan areas. However, after reading this chapter and becoming familiar with the equipment, software, and services listed, you should have a good idea of what you will have to buy, why you will need it, and what you will have to pay for it on the retail market.

Close to Home

There are obvious advantages in dealing with a single nearby company, but you may choose to do otherwise. The manager of your local Radio Shack store may be a real pill, and the owner of Computerama may be a medical management enthusiast who also offers all his products at 50 percent off. Or you may be a person who likes to shop around for everything and can put up with the heartache of an out-of-service printer shipped from Ashtabula. The point is that Radio Shack consistently meets the seven requirements for running a good operation; and it does so at a price about 50 percent less than the price of having them met by a consulting firm.

INSTRUCTION

It is possible to learn most of the prepackaged software programs by oneself. But the process can be tedious and not very efficient. Business operations will benefit from having secretaries rapidly learn major programs from professional instructors. All Radio Shack computer stores have an instructional component. They offer a number of courses, three of which will be particularly helpful to you and your staff in getting your system operational and working maximally.

Operator's Course

The operator's course runs about four hours and costs $50. You and your secretary (or computer operator) should take this course. The operator's course deals with fundamentals, such as how to turn the machine on and where to insert the disks. It is model oriented; that is, the course is designed for specific Radio Shack computers (Models II, 12, and 16). Taking the course would be of limited value if you own another computer. Among the topics covered in this course are: (1) introduction to microcomputers, (2) physical description of the machine, (3) diskettes, (4) backing up system and data diskettes, (5) running in BASIC, and (6) running application programs.

Word Processing Course

Scripsit is Radio Shack's word processing program. Definitely send your secretary to the Scripsit course. It is given on two consecutive days. The Scripsit manual contains an excellent, self-administered tutorial, including six audiocassettes. The problem with any tutorial is that unless large blocks of time are available, progress can be slow. However, after two days in this course plus a little practice, your secretary will become a whiz at word processing. The course costs $150 and is well worth it. Whether or not *you* take the course is optional. If you have time to fuss with the tutorial or want to ask your secretary how she moved a paragraph from page 1 to page 3, that's OK. If you're not going to type or your involvement with word processing will be limited to correcting misspelling, then skip the course.

Data Base Course

Profile is Radio Shack's data base management or information retrieval program. Because Profile is a universally used software package, you don't have to be a Radio Shack user to benefit from the course, although your version may have slight variations. It takes a full day, costs about $90, and is best taken by the individual in your office who will be in charge of computer operations. At its simplest level, Profile can be used for filing addresses of clients and then printing labels based on any configuration of demographic or personal characteristics that you might employ at any given time. PROFILE can be merged with word processing programs to produce personal letters to any number of selected individuals. For example, a Profile/Scripsit merge could be a personal letter to any patient owing more than $75 for more than 45 days. The program files may be combined to send out, say, 100 letters, each individually addressed, each indicating exactly how many days the account is overdue and how much the individual owes. After the base letter and sorting parameters have been defined, hundreds of personalized letters can be typed automatically on your letterhead with just one or two keystrokes.

EQUIPMENT

There are two types of equipment: (1) the basic system, consisting of a computer (CPU, VDT, keyboard, and disk drives) and a printer and (2) additional equipment, which usually includes such items as a modem, a printer tractor, and acoustic housing. All of these items are described below.

Computer

Radio Shack has two "top-of-the-line" computers, the Model 16 and the Model 12. The Model 16 has both an 8-bit and a 16-bit microprocessor. The Model 12 has only an eight-bit microprocessor. The difference in cost is $1,800. However, unless you plan a multi-user operation (more than one terminal connected to one CPU), the Model 12 will do everything the Model 16 can do for your office.

The Model 12 is aesthetically pleasing (see accompanying picture). A sleek, white cabinet houses the CPU. It has a high-resolution, 12-inch, green phosphorous monitor (CRT) and one to two thin-line, double-density, 8-inch floppy disk drives. The video display has upper- and lowercase characters and is 80 characters wide and 24 lines deep. The computer contains a Z-80A eight-bit microprocessor and supports 80K RAM. These figures are quite acceptable for single-user medical office systems. The video display is crisp, resulting in reduced eye fatigue.

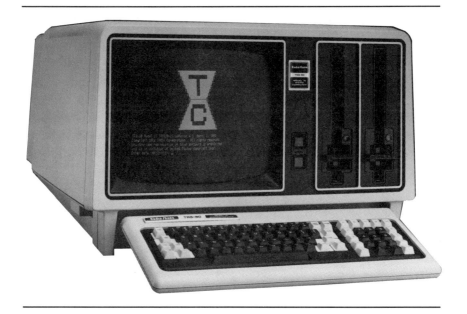

Keyboard

The keyboard is detachable, and it has a high-quality feel. It contains 82 keys, including a numeric pad. There are special keys for Hold, Caps, ESC, Break, CTRL, Repeat, and up/down/right/left arrows, plus eight programmable function keys (F1-F8). The numeric pad lacks operand keys (plus, minus, multiply, divide), requiring the user to go back to the typewriter pad. With the exception of this single minor inconvenience, the keyboard is intelligently laid out and easy to use.

Floppy Disk Drives

Each disk drive can store 1,250,000 characters in its double-sided, double-density mode. At present, ironically, most of the Radio Shack programs are written to operate more efficiently in the single-sided mode, thus greatly reducing the actual storage available.

Operating System

The operating systems are stored primarily on the diskettes and to a small extent in ROM. As all Radio Shack programs have the operating system already built into the diskette, it becomes loaded automatically whenever a program is booted into the computer. The Model 12 is fairly easy to use. Nonetheless, there are several utilities that will require study or instruction for the user to be able to operate with any facility. The rank novice may find the instructions for the Backup, Format, Copy, and Move utilities somewhat confusing.

There are two ways to go with the Model 12—by floppy disk drive or by hard disk drive. For guidelines on which to choose, see Chapter 4. If you choose floppy, then you will be using a two-disk drive system to support the Medical Office System software and to facilitate the making of backups. If you choose hard disk, then you will probably choose a Model 12 with only one disk drive. This will reduce the cost of the computer about $800, as only one floppy drive is necessary to back up a hard disk drive. There may be some inconvenience if you wish to make floppy backups of floppy application programs, though the need to do so would be infrequent.

Hard Disk Drive

The Model 12 requires some modification to be used with a hard disk drive. A $200 card cage will have to be installed by a Radio Shack technician at a cost of about $60. The Radio Shack primary hard disk system will store approximately 12 megabytes. This should be ample for almost any Medical Office System. The hard disk consists of six sealed platters that are unremovable. Once installed, this hard disk system is easy to use and will work up to

10 times as fast as floppy. It has an easy-to-use backup utility (Save and Restore) that transfers data in compressed form to double-sided, double-density floppy diskettes.

Printer

The choice will be be between two printers: the Daisy Wheel II and the DMP 2100. Both cost the same, nearly $2,000. The Daisy Wheel II produces impecable, letter-quality results at about 500 words a minute. The DMP 2100 can produce near-letter-quality results, and in certain modes it is four times as fast as the Daisy Wheel II. In the data processing (DP) mode it can produce 215 lines per minute of a 20-character column and 60 lines per minute of a 132-character column. In the correspondence mode it can produce 774 words a minute. We tested the Daisy Wheel II extensively and found it to be a workhorse that never failed. The quality of the results was as good as you will find anywhere. The Daisy Wheel II is one of the noisier printers, and it vibrates considerably. However, it can be placed in an attractive, self-contained acoustic shell that has its own fan for air circulation. The shell, which costs just under $400, renders it quite docile. The shell would be recommended if the printer is to be near any conversation area, including telephone. We did not test the DMP 2100 extensively, but in running it through its paces, we found it easy to use, relatively quiet, and versatile. It produced correspondence that would be acceptable to many practitioners.

Bidirectional Tractors

A tractor is recommended for the printer, especially to assist in long runs of billing and insurance forms (see Chapter 4). The DWII tractor costs $290, and the DMP2100 tractor costs $170.

Modem

A modem is necessary for any type of telephone communication. The Radio Shack direct-connect modem, which retails for $99, is easy to use and highly reliable. The auto-answer, auto-dial, direct-connect Modem II, which costs $249, is a bit more complicated to use and would be incorporated into a system that required receiving data at times when the computer might be unattended.

FURNITURE

This is one area in which practitioners are sometimes penny-wise and pound-foolish. Expensive equipment designed to increase efficiency is sometimes placed inconveniently in corners or on flimsy furniture. Cables and paper are run helter-skelter. Heavy-duty tables and desks, especially designed for microprocessing, are recommended. These tables will support vibrating printers and have places to direct cables and paper.

The Radio Shack system desk and printer stand are attractive and sturdy and complement each other. They come kicked down, but they are very easy to assemble. The printer stand accommodates both the DWII and the DMP2100 handily. The work station comes with an optional desk drawer and shelf that is handy for storing supplies, the hard disk drive, or the floppy expansion unit. The desk is the right depth for the Model 12 and leaves about 5 square feet of extra work space. The printer stand is rock sturdy and is just the right size. The stand costs $150; the system desk, $270; and the system desk drawer/shelf, $130.

SOFTWARE

Medical Office System

Radio Shack's MOS entry is inexpensive ($750); designed for Models II, 12, and 16; and provided with many special features. So well provided, in fact, that it is easier to describe by what it lacks than by what it has.[1]

    User Modification. Possibly the most important feature of the Radio Shack MOS is that it permits easy user modification of its insurance form program. It can be modified to print information in any configuration that the user wishes, on as many different forms as might practically be incorporated by a practice. Simple modifications can be made in about 10 minutes, and new forms can be designed from scratch in about four to five hours, with no

---

[1] The Radio Shack MOS does not schedule appointments, produce proof of posting, or keep a general ledger (or interact with one). These features are not critical, and their absence is greatly outweighed by the many features that the program does possess. The Radio Shack MOS is interactive with Radio Shack's word processing and data base management programs.

special training or skills. The program is also equipped with the latest of the most universally used insurance claim forms, that of the AMA.

Documentation. There are over 250 pages of documentation to lead the user through the MOS. The manual is well written and very helpful.

Capacity. The package will accommodate 10 physicians, 36 locations, 4 recall notes or medications per patient, 2 recall dates per patient, up to 2 insurance companies per patient, and 50 line items per invoice. In the hard disk mode the MOS will support 64,000 active patients and 64,000 transactions, which can include 999 procedures and 999 diagnoses.

Standard Forms. Statements are run on standard, off-the-shelf forms, as the program automatically prints the name of the practice and the return address. Dunning messages may be automatically printed on the forms. They may be folded once and placed in a double-windowed envelope, eliminating the need for either typing an address or using a preprinted envelope.

User Friendly. The Radio Shack MOS has an easy-to-use transaction mode, enabling charges to be billed by up to 10 doctors in multiple locations with as many as three responsible parties per patient (the patient plus two insurance companies). Write-offs and adjustments are no problem. Precedures, diagnoses, and fees may be automatically or manually entered.

Data Bases. The files house a wide range of demographic and practice information. The system has a built-in data base management program, permitting the sorting and listing of patients by 32 variables ranging from "amount owed" to "medication/date."

Financial Reports. The program has a detailed financial reporting system. It can produce several types of daily, monthly, and yearly reports on patient/insurance accounts and on the productivity of doctors and practice locations. It also has a graph mode for visual comparisons of financial data regarding practice productivity (see Figure 11–1).

FIGURE 11-1
Graphic Representation of Financial Transactions

```
                     M O N T H   A T   A   G L A N C E

                              For Month 01  Year 1984
           ..........................................................
$7,220    .00000                                                      .
$6,768    .00000                                                      .
$6,317    .00000 00000                                                .
$5,866    .00000 00000                                                .
$5,415    .00000 00000                                                .
$4,963    .00000 00000                                                .
$4,512    .00000 00000                                                .
$4,061    .00000 00000 00000                                          .
$3,610    .00000 00000 00000                                          .
$3,158    .00000 00000 00000                                          .
$2,707    .00000 00000 00000                                          .
$2,256    .00000 00000 00000 00000                                    .
$1,805    .00000 00000 00000 00000                                    .
$1,353    .00000 00000 00000 00000                                    .
  $902    .00000 00000 00000 00000                                    .
  $451    .00000 00000 00000 00000 00000 00000 00000                  .
   $0     .00000 00000 00000 00000 00000 00000 00000 00000 00000      .
           ..........................................................
           Total  New   Pat   Ins   Adj P Adj I Adj   A/R   Cash  Write
           Recpt  Charg Paym  Paym  Paym  Paym  Chrgs Due   In    Offs
```

Scripsit

Scripsit is Radio Shack's word processing program for Models II, 12, and 16. It has undergone a number of refinements and is considered by many to be the standard against which other programs in the field are compared. From a word processing standpoint, there is probably nothing that Scripsit cannot do. This powerful package costs $399. It produces a logical directory that permits the user to store, review, and retrieve documents with great ease. Many formats for page organization, printing, and editing are available. Scripsit features rapid text manipulation ranging from the simple addition and deletion of characters to complicated reorganizations of pages and the merging of multiple documents. User keys may be defined so that words and paragraphs can be stored and retrieved with a single keystroke. Scripsit has a number of global search modes by means of which words are instantly found and changed, either manually or automatically. It has a full range of print codes, including super- and subscript, underline, boldface, and margin justification.

A minor disadvantage of Scripsit is that it is a double-windowed program. Print codes are represented on the screen with graphic characters, so that the printed copy may vary visually from the screen copy. Most computer operators find this to be only a minor inconvenience because after using the program for a few weeks, the operator quickly interprets the print codes and sees the screen "mentally" as it will print out.[2]

Scripsit Spelling and Hyphenation Dictionary

This $199 program is a companion to Scripsit. It is a 150,000-word dictionary with room for 1,100 user-defined words. Once the dictionary has been installed, any document may be checked against it with only a keystroke. The searches are relatively rapid, usually only a few seconds per document. Words in the document that do not match against the dictionary are highlighted in the document itself. The user may either correct the spelling or pass over the word. A minor weakness of the program is that it does not provide alternative spelling prompts for the user. Its principal ad-

---

[2] Radio Shack has recently come out with a powerful word processing program especially designed for hard disk. This new program still has some "minor" bugs in its directory listing utility. It is anticipated that these relatively few problems, with this otherwise versatile program, will be rectified by the time this book is published.

vantage is that it is a huge dictionary. That means the identification of fewer false positives.

Profile Plus

It is a versatile program that can be adequately learned by the self-study tutorial provided in the manual (it requires about six hours to learn). Perhaps its only noticeable disadvantage is that it takes about 45 seconds to enter the "inquiry" mode in the floppy operating system and about 30 seconds in hard disk. The inquiry mode is the one that displays the various screens or "electronic filing cards." Once in the inquiry mode, it is possible to go from one "card" to another almost instantaneously. The irritating initial wait would be troublesome only if it were necessary to go in and out of the inquiry mode frequently during the course of the day. Apart from this minor disadvantage, the program is easy to master and provides a clean and efficient method for keeping track of names, addresses, and other variables. It permits handy printing of envelopes, labels, and specially designed reports. Profile is also interactive with Radio Shack's Medical Office System and Scripsit, permitting individualized letters to be sent to large groups of patients.

Visi-Calc

Visi-Calc is Radio Shack's single-user electronic spread sheet program. Figure 11–2 demonstrates a final balancing report of insurance billing. All tabulations are automatic, with the column on the right (true/false) providing immediate information regarding balancing status. This old standby is very versatile and has withstood years of testing. It is the program that reportedly put Apple on the map (not vice versa). Radio Shack is now also distributing Multi-Plan, a slightly more versatile spread sheet that lends itself to multi-user operations.

SUPPLIES

Somewhat surprising is the array of supplies needed to run a computer operation. The printer seems to dine on paper and ribbons. The archiving of disks may require purchasing these items by the carton. Special forms are often required for billing pro-

FIGURE 11-2
User Adapted Visi-Calc

PAGE 1   DAY SHEET PROOF   YEAR 83

INSURANCE BILLING

	Charge	Payment	NEW BAL	Pre Bal	PROOF	
1982	54035.76	55213.23	940784.06	941961.53	940784.06	TRUE
JAN	4338.22	4009.07	53121.00	52791.85	53121.00	TRUE
FEB	2240.61	4918.26	36147.35	38825.00	36147.35	TRUE
MAR	3910.34	2765.89	41753.40	40608.95	41753.40	TRUE
1ST QUART	10489.17	11693.22	131021.75	132225.80		
APR	4594.28	6455.48	53998.95	55860.15	53998.95	TRUE
MAY	5500.35	4161.75	60175.75	58837.15	60175.75	TRUE
JUNE	4616.00	6870.10	56928.55	59182.65	56928.55	TRUE
2ND QUART	14710.63	17487.33	171103.25	173879.95		
JUL	3536.54	7642.54	48287.40	52393.40	48287.40	TRUE
AUG	3951.26	4779.60	37684.61	38512.95	37684.61	TRUE
SEP	3050.72	5867.38	39576.18	42392.84	39576.18	TRUE
3RD QUART	10538.52	18289.52	125548.19	133299.19		
OCT	635.77	4567.52	17520.75	21452.50	17520.75	TRUE
NOV	963.89	1033.59	17569.66	17639.36	17569.66	TRUE
DEC	2581.12	3806.82	36285.25	37510.95	36285.25	TRUE
4TH QUART	4180.78	9407.93	71375.66	76602.81		
YEAR TOT	39919.10	56878.00	499048.85	516007.75		

grams. Fear not—Radio Shack has not neglected this fertile source of income. At the end of this chapter is a listing of almost all the supply items you will need to get started and keep going for the first 6 to 12 months.

AVOIDING DOWNTIME

Service

Most of the items discussed here are fully guaranteed for 90 days. If the equipment fails, it may be brought to any Radio Shack store, from which it will be transferred to a Radio Shack computer center for repair. Most repairs may be made overnight.

Service Contracts

What happens after 90 days? Most problems will surface soon after a system is bought (if they surface at all), but some problems may take a while to develop, particularly the "bad connection" variety. Since even simple repairs tend to be costly, some consideration should be given to an extended warranty or to a warranty that will include on-site service.

Maintenance

Although some warranties include periodic cleaning and maintenance, this is definitely a do-it-yourself item. Regular use of dustcovers is the cheapest and most effective maintenance procedure available. Apart from careful cleaning of the CRT and vacuuming of the computer, keyboard, disk drives, printer, and surrounding areas, there are only two other cleaning jobs, both of which may be done in seconds with the help of a floppy disk drive cleaning kit and a Daisy Wheel cleaning kit.

Support

Last, but certainly not least, is support. Support is synonymous with "Help!" It is what you need when "it doesn't work" or "I can't figure it out." Radio Shack offers a six-level support system: (1) sales personnel, (2) instructors, (3) hotline service, (4) program registration and update, (5) service department, and (6) newsletter.

When Things Go Haywire

The first line of defense is a call to the computer center with questions directed to the sales or service staff and instructors. The members of the sales and service staff are most familiar with equipment problems; the instructors are most familiar with software problems. If they cannot come up with the answer, then Radio Shack has a series of telephone numbers in Texas, manned by folks who do nothing but troubleshoot. The numbers are often busy in the afternoon and are not toll-free. However, once the problem has been defined by you and researched there, the answer is precise. Figure on a 15- to 30-minute long-distance bill; not a bad deal for that kind of advice.

Radio Shack updates its programs with patches and, in some cases, new program disks. Updates are secured by mailing in a registration card when software is purchased. Finally, Radio Shack publishes a monthly periodical, *TRS-80 Microcomputer News*. It is mailed free for the first 12 months after the purchase of a Radio Shack computer. It contains information about how to get the most efficient use of the equipment and software. Customer columns and letters are replete with helpful hints and homemade programs.

THE SHOPPING LIST

As indicated at the beginning of this chapter, the Radio Shack catalog is an excellent reference for determining the price and description of probably every item needed to run a computerized office. The accompanying list will enable the practitioner to implement a complete, high-quality, single-user computer system. All of the items listed are from Radio Shack Computer Catalog RSC11. They are given here for information only: to assist the practitioner in understanding what kinds of equipment, supplies, software, and support are needed to computerize the office management of a medical, dental, or psychological practice. Prices may vary, and individual needs may dictate a different manufacturer or more or less equipment. Although the list does not represent an endorsement of the items, all have been personally tested and have been found to be of excellent quality and service and highly adaptable to the needs of most practices.

	Cat. No.	Floppy	Hard
Basic hardware			
One-disk TRS-80 Model 12 computer	26-4004	—	$ 2,799.00
Two-disk TRS-80 Model 12 computer	26-4005	3,499.00	—
Primary hard disk drive	26-5263	—	2,999.00
Model 12 card cage	26-6017	—	199.00
Daisywheel II printer	26-1158	1,995.00	1,995.00
Bidirectional tractor feed	26-1447	289.95	289.95
6-foot parallel printer cable	26-4401	39.00	39.00
Subtotal		5,822.95	8,350.95
Communications hardware			
Direct-connect modem	26-1172	99.00	99.00
RS-232C serial interface 5-foot cable	26-4403	39.95	39.95
Subtotal		138.95	138.95
Furniture			
Custom work station (system desk)	26-4303	269.95	269.95
Printer stand	26-4305	149.95	249.95
System drawer	26-4304	—	129.95
Work station chair	74-1057	199.95	199.95
Subtotal		619.85	849.80
Maintenance and static control			
Universal 8-inch disk drive cleaning kit	26-4909	29.95	29.95
Daisy Wheel printwheel cleaning kit	26-1320	16.95	16.95
Antistatic spray	26-515	5.95	5.95
Screen cleaner	26-1318	2.95	2.95
Model 12 dustcover	26-526	9.95	9.95
Daisy Wheel II and tractor dustcover	26-516	7.95	7.95
Antistatic mat	70-500	79.95	79.95
Subtotal		153.65	153.65
Software			
Medical Office System	26-4508	750.00	750.00
Scripsit (word processing) for 8-inch floppy	26-4531	399.00	—
Scripsit (word processing) for hard disk	26-4835	—	399.00
Profile Plus (data base)	26-4515	299.00	299.00
Visi-Calc Enhanced (spread sheet)	26-4521	299.00	299.00
Videotex (communication software)	26-2221	29.95	29.95
Subtotal		1,776.95	1,776.95
Courses			
Model 12 operating system		69.95	—
with 12-megabyte hard disk		—	99.95
Scripsit (word processing) (Model 12)		149.95	149.95
Subtotal		212.90	212.90

	Cat. No.	Floppy	Hard
Supplies (6 to 12 months)			
14⅞ × 11-inch one-part greenbar, 3,500 sheets	26–1417	49.95	49.95
9½ × 11-inch one-part greenbar, 3,500 sheets	26–1463	39.95	39.95
General-purpose form, 1,000 sheets	72–219	25.00	25.00
Blank envelopes (billing), 1,000	72–206	45.00	45.00
One-wide, Fanfold mailing labels, 4,000	26–1404	19.95	19.95
14⅞ × 11-inch hanging binders, quantity 10	70–505	34.95	34.95
11 × 8½-inch hanging binders, quantity 10	70–506	34.95	34.95
DWII carbon film cartridges (multistrike), 4 cartons (3 per)	26–1419	12/84.00	12/84.00
DWII nylon ribbon cartridges, 3 cartons	26–1449	3/32.85	3/32.85
8-inch SSDD unformated diskette, 3 packages (10 per)	26–4906	3/179.85	—
8-inch DSDD unformated diskette, 3 packages (10 per)	26–4960	—	3/209.85
Subtotal		546.45	576.45
Accessories			
8-inch diskette boxes, quantity 3 to 5	26–4956	5/29.75	3/17.85
8-inch diskette file box, quantity 1	26–4953	39.95	—
14⅞-inch stacking data tray, quantity 3	26–1309	3/25.47	3/25.47
Printview ruler, quantity 1	26–1313	2.95	2.95
8-inch diskette replacement labels, package of 50	26–4955	1.95	1.95
Extra print wheel (Prestige Elite, 12 pitch)	26–1421	29.95	29.95
Automatic power strip	26–1429	69.95	69.95
Antiglare panel	26–1457	29.95	29.95
Subtotal		229.92	178.07
Nice to have, but not essential			
Scripsit spelling and hypenation dictionary			
For floppy	26–4534	199.00	—
For hard	26–4434	—	199.00
General ledger (accounting software)	26–4501	199.00	199.00
Paper caddy	74–551	79.95	79.95
Subtotal		477.95	477.95
Courses, nice to have, but not essential			
Profile Plus (Model 12)		99.95	99.95
Visi-Calc (Model 12)		89.95	89.95
Subtotal		189.90	189.90
Totals (with extra items)		$10,169.47	$12,875.57
Totals (with only essential items)		$ 9,501.62	$12,207.72

Note: Prices may vary from store to store and are subject to change.
Source: Radio Shack Catalog RSC11, Radio Shack/Tandy Corp., 1984.

Chapter 12
Alternatives to the Computer

ALTERNATIVES
ADVANTAGES
   Investment
   Broader Programs
   Freedom from Troubleshooting
   Cost Containment
   Staff Training
DISADVANTAGES
   Lack of Spontaneity
   Program Modification and Development
   Insurance Statements
   Word Processing

ALTERNATIVES

It is not necessary to own a computer to enjoy the benefits of one. There are companies that provide complete services based on information collected on the usual day sheet employed in a practice (see Figure 12–1). The practitioner's office staff handles transactions in the customary way; that is, payment is taken and a receipt is given utilizing a one-write system. One pioneer of this system is Safeguard Business Systems, Inc. Its system permits the practitioner to make an entry on a day sheet, patient ledger card, and transaction slip (receipt) in one quick step through the use of NCR paper (makes carbons without carbon paper), specially designed forms, and a pegboard. This system has gone a long way toward modernizing medical and dental offices and is utilized in

FIGURE 12–1
Day Sheet

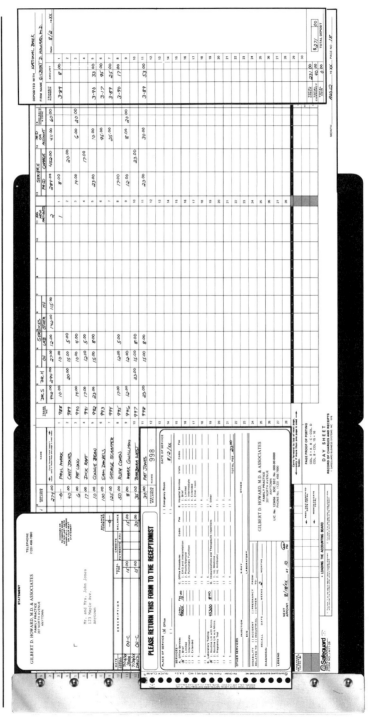

Reprinted with permission from Safeguard Business Systems, Inc.

most practices where more than five patients a week are seen. Several companies, including Safeguard, have adapted this system to produce long-distance data processing especially tailored to private practitioners in the allied health professions. It works roughly as follows.

Dr. Long is an orthopedic surgeon who provides about 25 consultations a day. With other transactions (e.g., payments received on account), these nearly fill one day sheet. Each Friday his secretary mails five day sheets to a nearby Safeguard office. A week later she receives a packet and a weekly financial and management report. Depending on the time of the month or year, the packet might contain completed patient billing statements or monthly or yearly financial status reports. The monthly reports consist of a missed payment report, a practice management summary report, a monthly recall listing, and an accounts receivable ledger. The weekly reports consist of recall notices, a day sheet summary report, an activity rejection report, a new accounts (changes and deletions) report, and an insurance report. In addition, Dr. Long receives quarterly and annual reports summarizing similar information (see Figures 12–2 and 12–3, refer to Appendix A for additional sample reports). Dr. Long pays a small monthly charge plus a per item charge of between $0.07 and $0.25 per account serviced each week or month. For the above services he pays approximately $175 monthly, depending on his actual usage.

ADVANTAGES

Investment

Use of an external computer system does not involve any capital investment, save possibly the very small investment in a pegboard system.

Broader Programs

Of course, computer bureau services utilize large mainframe computers. The more complex programs of these computers are able to generate more detailing of reports than can be generated by a microcomputer. Patient statements, for example, might include one of several levels of finance charges.

FIGURE 12–2
Missed Payment Report

```
 6/30/83   9:06 AM                               MEDICAL DEMONSTRATION                                               Page   1
Doc  1: JOHN J JONES MD                          MISSED PAYMENTS REPORT                                  MONTH END FOR JUN 83
 REF    FAMILY     FAMILY         FAMILY       INSURANCE  PREV    CURRENT   CURRENT   CURRENT     OVER      OVER      OVER PRACTICE
 MES      ID     LAST NAME      FIRST NAME MI LIABILITY  BAL     CHARGES   PAYMENTS  ADJ'S     30 DAYS   60 DAYS   90 DAYS END BAL
STMC    WORK PHONE      HOME PHONE                                                   DOC       OVER      OVER      OVER    DOCTOR
   LPD & AMOUNT     CONT AMT DUE      INS PAY                                       CURRENT   30 DAYS   60 DAYS   90 DAYS BALANCE


DR. SM ABBOT    ABBOT           THOMAS     T.     0.00      0.00    205.00    115.00      0.00      0.00      0.00      0.00     90.00
      125-5600-X52    320-5210                                                           90.00      0.00      0.00      0.0C     90.00
 -none-      0.00            0.00       115.00

       BENNETT  BENNETT         RICHARD           0.00    120.00    165.00    210.00     -5.00      0.00      0.00      0.0C     70.00
                      435-3535                                                            35.00      0.00      0.00      0.00     35.00
 -none-      0.00            0.00       210.00

       BLASS    BLASS           THOMAS     M.    25.20      0.00     45.00      0.00      0.00      0.00      0.00      0.00     45.00
                      567-5555                                                            45.00      0.00      0.00      0.00     45.00
 -none-      0.00            0.00         0.00

       CABOT    CABOT           JOHN              0.00     75.00    100.00    113.00     -7.00      0.00      0.00      0.00     55.00
      456-7777        456-7777                                                            55.00      0.00      0.00      0.00     55.00
 -none-      0.00            0.00       113.00

       WISH     WISH            FRANCES    G.    56.00      0.00    100.00      0.00      0.00      0.00      0.00      0.00    100.00
1                     555-5555                                                           100.00      0.00      0.00      0.00    100.00
 -none-      0.00            0.00         0.00
---------------------------------------------------------------------------------------------------------------------------------------

PRACTICE TOTALS:                                 81.20              615.00              -12.00                0.00               360.00
             0.00            0.00       438.00            195.00              438.00               0.00                0.00

DOCTOR TOTALS:                                                                          325.00                0.00               325.00
                                                                                                   0.00                0.00
```

FIGURE 12-3
Aged Receivables Report

```
6/30/83  9:06 AM                        MEDICAL DEMONSTRATION                                                    Page  1
Doc 1: JOHN J JONES  MD                 AGED RECEIVABLES REPORT                          MONTH END FOR JUN 83

REF   FAMILY  FAMILY       FAMILY           INSURANCE  PREV    CURRENT  CURRENT   CURRENT   OVER     OVER     OVER     OVER PRACTICE
MES    ID     LAST NAME    FIRST NAME MI    LIABILITY  BAL     CHARGES  PAYMENTS  ADJ'S     30 DAYS  60 DAYS  90 DAYS  END BAL
                                                                                  DOC       OVER     OVER     OVER     OVER DOCTOR
                                                                                  CURRENT   30 DAYS  60 DAYS  90 DAYS  BALANCE

DR. SM ABBOT   ABBOT       THOMAS      T.     0.00      0.00    205.00   115.00     0.00     0.00     0.00     0.00     90.00
                                                                                   90.00     0.00     0.00     0.00     90.00

TENNIS ACE     ACE         FRANCES            0.00     75.00    332.00   188.80   -17.20     0.00     0.00     0.00    201.00
                                                                                   67.55     0.00     0.00     0.00     67.55

BENNETT        BENNETT     RICHARD            0.00    120.00    165.00   210.00    -5.00     0.00     0.00     0.00     70.00
                                                                                   35.00     0.00     0.00     0.00     35.00

BLASS          BLASS       THOMAS      M.    25.20      0.00     45.00     0.00     0.00     0.00     0.00     0.00     45.00
                                                                                   45.00     0.00     0.00     0.00     45.00

CABOT          CABOT       JOHN               0.00     75.00    100.00   113.00    -7.00     0.00     0.00     0.00     55.00
                                                                                   55.00     0.00     0.00     0.00     55.00

CARD           CARD        JAMES              0.00     25.00     30.00    25.00     0.00     0.00     0.00     0.00     30.00
                                                                                   30.00     0.00     0.00     0.00     30.00

CASS           CASS        JAMES              0.00    112.00    136.68    48.68     0.00     0.00     0.00    63.32    200.00
                                                                                  106.68     0.00     0.00    63.32    170.00

GOLF   CLUB    CLUB        PATRICK            0.00      0.00    301.00   265.00     0.00     0.00     0.00     0.00     36.00
                                                                                   20.58     0.00     0.00     0.00     20.58

CARDS  HEART   HEART       MARY               0.00     45.00    365.00    75.00     0.00     0.00     0.00     0.00    335.00
                                                                                  308.37     0.00     0.00     0.00    308.37

PARKER         PARKER      JOHN               0.00    175.00    154.00   234.50     0.00     0.00     0.00     0.00     94.50
                                                                                   21.89     0.00     0.00     0.00     21.89

QUEEN          QUEEN       KATHLEEN          72.80     33.00    275.00   160.00    -8.00     0.00     0.00     0.00    140.00
                                                                                   27.96     0.00     0.00     0.00     27.96

WISH           WISH        FRANCES     G.    56.00      0.00    100.00     0.00     0.00     0.00     0.00     0.00    100.00
                                                                                  100.00     0.00     0.00     0.00    100.00
                                           ------   -------  --------  -------   -------   -----    -----    -----   --------
PRACTICE TOTALS:                            154.00    660.00   2208.68  1434.98   -37.20     0.00     0.00    63.32    1396.50

DOCTOR TOTALS:                                                                    908.03     0.00     0.00    63.32     971.35

                            * DENOTES (   0) FAMILIES WITH CONTRACT BALANCES DUE
```

Freedom from Troubleshooting

The practitioner is spared all the headaches involved in the production of reports and statements. The following problems no longer create havoc: power failures, failure to understand the manual, printer failures, and the myriad other problems that can slow down or halt a computer operation.

Cost Containment

Fees are based on use. There is no need for maintenance contracts and computer supply orders (ribbon, diskettes, etc.) to keep the computer up and running.

Staff Training

No new skills are needed. All computer technology is taken care of by the service provider.

DISADVANTAGES

Lack of Spontaneity

On-the-spot reports cannot be produced. The practitioner must wait to receive the weekly, monthly, or quarterly reports. The turnaround time will usually be six business days. The same turnaround time is required for corrections and adjustments to patient financial records.

Program Modification and Development

Cost containment is achieved by using whatever programs and services are "on the shelf" and made available to you by the service provider. There is little or no opportunity to modify or develop a program especially for your practice.

Insurance Statements

Most service providers will provide a status report regarding insurance payments but will not provide the actual insurance billing statement. The reason is that the various third-party payers require different forms and information. Such differences do not lend themselves well to service bureau use.

Word Processing

The services provided are limited to financial management. Such options as word processing and telecommunication are not available.

A contract with a computer service bureau can be an excellent interim step for a practitioner contemplating embarking on computerization. The initial costs are minuscule as compared with the cost of obtaining equipment. Use of a service bureau will permit the practitioner to organize her office toward computerization. Once this has been done, the option of purchasing a computer can always be exercised.

Chapter 13
Helping the Computer Make Money for You

THE COMPUTER CAN MAKE MONEY FOR YOU
OPTIMAL USE
STIMULATING PATIENT/CLIENT INTEREST
    Recall
    Follow-up
    Letters to Referral Sources
    Mailings to Potential Referral Sources
BILLING AND COLLECTION
    Billing Dates and Procedures
    Tracking Accounts
ANCILLARY USE OF THE COMPUTER

THE COMPUTER CAN MAKE MONEY FOR YOU

As you have seen, the computer will require a great deal of attention. Either the practitioner or an employee will spend many extra hours in learning how to operate the computer system and keep it going. At some point the learning and maintenance will reach an optimal level. The software packages have been mastered; you've discovered, quite by accident, an undocumented word processing command to hyphenate your text; a colleague tells you how to make your financial spread sheets calculate faster; the company finally informs you of a patch that successfully debugs your data base management system. Now the time has come to have the computer make money for *you*—to put effort into having the computer generate business and enhanced cash flow.

There are two ways in which the computer can make money for you. It can be used to stimulate patient/client interest and referral, and it can be used to augment billing and collection.

OPTIMAL USE

To use the computer optimally, it is essential that programs be interactive, particularly accounts receivable, data base management, and word processing. Interaction permits program merging. Most MOS programs provide for the flagging or sorting of patients on a large number of fields. In addition, there are usually two or more user fields for the storage of any type of information that the practitioner may wish to include. Generally, these fields are used for medication tracking and recall, which are particularly adaptable to reaching or communicating with patients who fall into certain categories. In addition, most MOS programs will automatically indicate "date last seen" in a separate field. Given the above conditions, the following methods may be utilized to stimulate a practice.

STIMULATING PATIENT/CLIENT INTEREST

Recall

This system is most frequently used in dentistry. The computer is asked to search for anyone not seen in six or seven months. These patients are flagged, and the following may be produced: (1) Labels, which are affixed to either postcards or envelopes containing a message stating that six months have gone by since the last checkup and encouraging the patient to call. (2) Personalized merged letters to patients, reminding them to come in, which are produced by merging the names and addresses of flagged patients with the word processing program. A more aggressive practitioner might tie these personalized letters to an appointment program, actually setting the appointment time for the patient and encouraging the patient to call if the time is inconvenient. A personal follow-up letter to these and other patients scheduled to come in the following week may be used to more efficiently reduce no-shows.

Follow-up

Patients often appreciate letters of inquiry from the practitioner. The following letter and questionnaire are an example of a merge of word processing and MOS by a practitioner providing services in hypnosis. The words in braces { } identify data variables and are used to extract precise information from patients' files.

The responses enable the doctor to update her methods, and the letters themselves serve to stimulate patients who want to return or to refer someone else.

FIGURE 13–1
Sample Merge Letter to Patient

{DATE}

Ms. {FIRST} {LAST}
{ADDRESS}
{CITY} {STATE} {ZIP}

Dear Ms. {LAST}:

I hope that you have been successful in dealing with the {TYPE} issue and that learning self-hypnosis has been helpful. When you were seen in {SEEN}, I mentioned that I would be contacting you to find out how you were doing. Would you take a moment to fill out and return the enclosed form. It will not only let me know about you specifically but will also be of great value to me in updating the hypnosis program.

Sometimes people like to return for a follow-up visit after six months. If you would like to do so, just call.

Sincerely,

Barbara McDonald, Ph.D.

Enclosures

FIGURE 13-2
Accompanying Merge Questionnaire

HYPNOSIS QUESTIONNAIRE

Name: {FIRST} {LAST}
Month seen: {SEEN}
Type of hypnosis: Single session for {TYPE}

Check the answer that best describes you.

Answer the next question only if you came for smoking.

1. a. I don't smoke.
   b. I smoke less.
   c. I smoke the same.
   d. I smoke more.

Answer the next question only if you came for weight.

2. a. I weigh much less.
   b. I weigh somewhat less.
   c. I weigh about the same.
   d. I weigh more.

Answer the next question only if you came for pain.

3. a. I hurt much less.
   b. I hurt somewhat less.
   c. I hurt about the same.
   d. I hurt more.

Answer all the questions below.

4. a. Self-hypnosis helped a lot.
   b. It helped some.
   c. It helped just a little.
   d. It didn't help.

5. I would return again for hypnosis: _____ Yes _____ No
   Why?

6. I would recommend hypnosis to a friend: _____ Yes _____ No
   Why?

7. Comments:

Please return questionnaire in enclosed envelope.

Letters to Referral Sources

Keeping fresh in the minds of individuals who refer helps to keep one's practice lively. Many practitioners like to send periodic letters to referral sources. The computer simplifies the process of determining when such a letter was last sent. In the place reserved for medication/dates, one might put RFU840515, which would indicate that a Referral Follow-Up letter was last sent on 5/15/84. Weekly or monthly, the practitioner may use the computer to search the files and quickly produce a list older than 180 days.

Mailings to Potential Referral Sources

Most MOS packages provide for the recording of the patient's address but not for the recording of the referring doctor's address. Moreover, MOS packages do not provide for a general listing of vendors or other individuals who are service providers or potential

FIGURE 13-3
Master File, Screen I

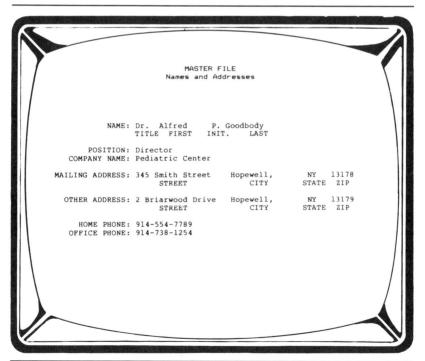

FIGURE 13–4
Master File, Screen II

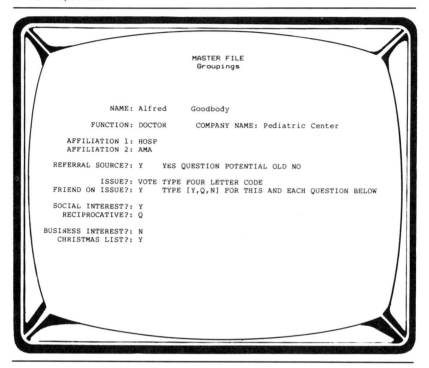

referral sources. Such listings are typically stored in data base management programs (see Chapter 14). These software packages are easily modifiable by the practitioner. The accompanying three-screen program, used by one practitioner, is designed to sort on the variables listed therein. The division into three screens has been made only for visual clarity. All of the information could have been placed on one screen. With this program it is possible for the practitioner to produce labels, lists, and word processing merges on any of the variables listed.

There are many things that can be done with the data base indicated on the screens. The most crucial advantage is that the practitioner can define categories of potential referents and communicate with them through the mail with less effort than has previously been possible. Here are some examples:

1. A label can be printed for each person marked Y, or "yes," on the variable called "Christmas list" to generate labels for a season's greetings mailing.

FIGURE 13–5
Master File, Screen III

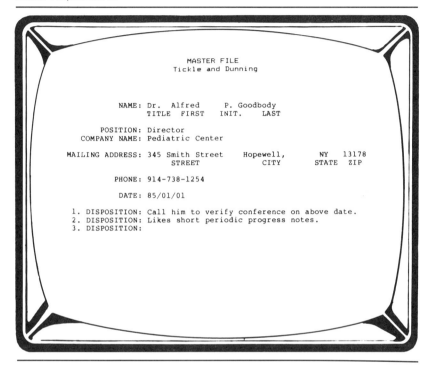

2. Since the computer can quickly sort many details, it is possible to generate a very specific list based on some combination of specified variables. For example, an oncologist may wish to send out a notice of a program or services to people in one of the following categories:

Function: Clergy or Psychotherapist.
Affiliation: Hospice, Inc., or City Hospital.

Data base systems are not difficult to design with the help of off-the-shelf software packages. However, initial information must be entered into the computer. A list of 300 or more names, addresses, and variables will take a while to develop and record. Once this has been done, the work becomes relatively easy. Again, the computer does not save work initially. Its strength lies in quick execution of these tedious, repetitive steps—sorting and duplicating.

BILLING AND COLLECTION

Billing Dates and Procedures

It is an old adage that if you wish to be paid promptly, you must bill promptly and accurately. If used properly, the computer can facilitate billing and other procedures related to the collection of fees. Naturally, no system is more effective than being paid the full fee at the time of service delivery. But the times being what they are, the probability is that the practitioner will be tied in some way to insurance companies or will have a number of patients who ask to be billed on a monthly payment plan.

Once a system is fully installed, most MOS packages will make the billing procedure about five times as fast as doing it by hand. A secretary/bookkeeper takes about five business days to get out insurance and patient statements for the average practice with a once-a-month billing cycle. With a computer the same procedure would take about eight hours. If the practice requires a full-time clerk to do billing, then the alphabet is often divided into equal quarters and billing begins on the first day of each week for a quarter. Without the computer, usually a week is spent on each quarter; with the computer, only a day per week is spent. The time freed up can then be used for other activities related to collection and the promotion of better cash flow, as indicated below.

Tracking Accounts

Because the computer so readily handles tedious chores, it is possible (and desirable) to develop and maintain an understandable and well-thought-out computerized system of collecting. Most MOS packages provide detailed reporting of accounts receivable and account status. Most important is the calculation of the ages of invoices; that is, what portion of an account is, for example, 30 days old or 60, 90, or more than 120 days old. (See Figures 12–2 and 12–3.) Similar aging may be done for insurance companies, say, after 45 days. (Everybody knows that insurance companies are slow.) If you wish, the MOS will print automatic messages on bills to patients and insurance companies that are late in payment. This is a passive system that requires very little maintenance but it will work only if the practitioner takes the time to enter these messages entered into the computer.

It is best to develop policies with regard to what will be done with patients whose accounts fall into various age and amount classifications. The practitioner may wish to meet with the clerk on a weekly basis in order to look over the accounts receivable report and provide guidance. Accounts that are 30 days old might receive a personal merge letter; accounts that are 60 days old might receive a telephone call.

The power of the MOS lies in its ability to quickly and succinctly report the complete status of all accounts receivable. Gone are the days of having to search through a pile of account cards in an attempt to calculate the ages of various outstanding balances. In a large practice it is possible to routinely send out messages, personal or otherwise, to patients having any configuration of balance and age. For example, the following letter might be sent to all patients with a balance of more than $50 for more than 60 days.

{DATE}

{TITLE} {FIRST} {LAST}
{ADDRESS}
{CITY} {STATE} {ZIP}

Dear {TITLE} {LAST}:

Re: {BALANCE} Due

We did not receive a payment from you in {AGE} days. Your account has a current balance of {BALANCE}.
We would appreciate your putting a check in the mail for the full amount. If you have any questions, please call the office.

Sincerely,

Alfred P. Goodbody, M.D.

The final product requires a few keystrokes, plus loading the correct paper into the printer. All patient information and the boilerplate letter will already be in the computer.

ANCILLARY USE OF THE COMPUTER

The computer may be used to give and administer tests. The field of psychology probably makes greater use of the computer for these purposes than does any other. About two dozen psychological tests have been formatted to be given interactively between the patient and the computer (see Appendix D for example). In addition, the computer may be used to score and interpret these tests and produce a written narrative. Heretofore, practitioners, including psychologists, have often had to send patients in need of psychological testing to persons specialized in this procedure. Now it is possible for the practitioner to have psychological tests performed in her own office, obtain results immediately, and retain the income for this service. Of late, a number of companies have emerged in the computer-assisted psychological testing field. National Computer Systems (NCS) acquired the Psychometer from Compu-Psych, Inc.; the Psychometer is a self-contained portable unit with a special keyboard to make it very patient friendly. NCS also has a teleprocessing service called Arion. With it, the doctor can transmit test responses to the NCS computer, which tabulates the responses and transmits the results back to the doctor's computer. Arion is able to instantly provide scores, profiles, *and* interpretive reports. A principal advantage of Arion is that, with it, the doctor can offer a wide range of computer-analyzed psychological tests without having to make a large initial investment in elaborate equipment or programs. Chapter 14 provides more information about utilizing this type of external data base.

PsychSystems offers an array of psychological tests that can be given through multiple remote terminals. The tests can be scored, integrated, and interpreted by one of the new generations of small "mainframe" computers. Other companies are now providing reasonably priced software packages that permit the private practitioner to utilize her own equipment to score and interpret some of the more popular psychological tests.

Not all of the problems have been ironed out in this endeavor.

Complaints regarding paradoxes in the interpretive narratives still occur. One psychologist noted that he had administered a series of tests to a patient who had held 10 jobs in the past six months, only to find the narrative indicating that the patient "has qualities that are likely to result in a good work record." Although some of the tests used, such as the MMPI, have been around for a long time, others are relatively new and validation studies are still in the works. Some of the larger companies, such as NCS, have endeavoured to aggressively tackle this problem. To monitor clinical validity, NCS has aligned itself with the Univerity of Minnesota and has also secured the services of several well-published research psychologists. No doubt, in a few years these problems also will be dealt with by other companies. But in the meantime, the practitioner should be cautioned that in their present state the computerized psychological testing programs are not a substitute for the clinician's judgment. This leads us to a second problem area.

The existing law in most states is inadequate to encompass some of the ramifications of computerized psychological testing. In many cases, the safeguards are insufficient to ensure that the computers are operated by suitably trained individuals. Thus, the possibility arises that a wide variety of "psychological services" in the diagnostic field may fall into the hands of entrepreneurs rather than clinicians.

It is difficult to know whether or not the ethical issues involved will be addressed as rapidly as the technical issues. But it is probably fair to say that the questions regarding the validity of computerized tests will be answered within the next few years. Other fields besides psychology will be affected. One of the oldest patient-interactive programs has been utilized by hospitals in acquiring patient histories. Such programs have been refined to provide diagnostic hypotheses regarding patients. Most professional fields have had computer programs designed to assist them in the delivery of services. Accountants, lawyers, and brokers, for example, have been able to employ information retrieval systems and other programs to help in the analysis of their work. So long as a profession maintains control over the computer programs, the practitioners appear to be happy and even excited. It is when the programs fall into the hands of the "untrained" that the practitioners begin to feel threatened.

Chapter 14
My Name Is Fink
And What Do You Think,
I Sell Suits for Nothing;
or
How to Get Fitted for
Data Base Management
without Losing Your Shirt

MY NAME IS FINK
HOW DOES IT WORK?
DATA BASES
    Who's Who in the Zoo
    Recreational Data Base
READABLE DATA BASES
    Serious Data Bases
    Time and Charges
    Efficiency
    The Future

MY NAME IS FINK

There is a story about a man walking in the garment district in New York City. He becomes intrigued by a sign prominently displayed in a tailor shop window. It announces, "My name is Fink, and what do you think, I sell suits for nothing."

He goes in, and introduces himself to Mr. Fink. "Is that sign correct?" he asks.

"Absolutely!" Fink assures him.

"Well, measure me for a three-piece suit."

A week later the man comes to pick up his suit, but Mr. Fink also hands him a bill for $650.

In shock, the man points to the sign and says, "I don't understand. The sign says, 'My name is Fink, and what do you think, I sell suits for nothing!!!' "

Mr. Fink replies, "I'm sorry mister, you read the sign wrong. It says, 'My name is Fink, and what do you think, I sell suits for nothing???' "

It's a matter of inflection and orientation. All of this brings us to the Dow Jones Free Text Search, which isn't free. If you haven't already noticed, Dow Jones is the parent company of the publisher of this book, and if it will permit these few paragraphs to be printed, you will know how beneficient and good-humored it really is. The Dow Jones Free Text Search is one of more than a hundred data bases that are available to consumers who are willing to subscribe and pay for their use. In this data base, key words aren't needed to make a search. So, it's free text—you can use almost any word, at $1.20 a minute.

A data base or information retrieval system is a large compendium of information organized in a manner that permits access by key words or commands. The more up-to-date the data base, the easier it is to access, and the more relevant it is to the consumer's need, the greater is its value.

HOW DOES IT WORK?

The practitioner's computer becomes converted into a dumb terminal and is connected through the telephone lines to a mainframe computer housing the data base. This is done by means of a modem (a telephone interconnecting device) and a simple program that usually costs under $20. The different data bases are reached by first calling the number of a company or network that does nothing but interconnect to the data bases. Think of these as little Ma Bells or Sprints. One such company is Telenet. It has access numbers that are available in most major U.S. cities.

The routine goes something like this. Dr. Henry wishes to check up on the status of his stocks and bonds. On the main menu he presses V to bring up Videotex. In his town he dials 272-1800 to access Telenet, the "host" system telephone number. He then hears a high-pitched tone coming over the telephone receiver. He flicks a switch on the modem, hangs up the telephone, and receives prompts from Telenet on his CRT. The first one is, "Please type your terminal identifier." Dr. Henry has an A terminal, so he types A(ENTER). Next he is asked, "Please log in." He types "DOW1;;" without (ENTER).

He is asked, "What service, please???"

He responds, "DJNS."

He is asked to "Enter password," which he does.

The password is verified, and he is asked to enter his request.

He wishes to check on his Tandy stock. He types ",TAN" and, *voilà*, he sees the following on his screen:

STOCK	TAN
BID/CLOSE	49¾
ASKED/OPEN	49½
HIGH	50
LOW	48⅝
LAST	49⅜
VOLUME (100'S)	2776

He checks a few more quotes, gets a financial listing of another company, signs off, and returns to his customary duties.

DATA BASES

Who's Who in the Zoo

In 1981 the American Society for Information Science published a compendium called *Computer Readable Data Bases*. It lists over 500 data base systems, most of which are accessible from anywhere in the United States by anyone having a modest computer configuration. The two most popular systems are CompuServe and the Dow Jones News Retrieval Service (DJ/N). Like most others, these two data bases contain multiple bases. For example, once you access DJ/N, you may also elect to access its encyclopedia data base or its financial data bases. Some data bases are actually sent to the practitioner through the mail in the form of disks. The information is then transferred and stored in the practitioner's computer system. It's like a "disk of the month club." This gives the practitioner unlimited access to the disk without surcharges for each use. Unfortunately, however, even a double-sided, double-density 8-inch disk can deliver only about 1.2 million bytes of information. This may seem like a lot, but in the world of data base management it is very little.

Recreational Data Base

CompuServe and The Source are recreational in orientation. Although they provide opportunities for the acquisition of rather serious information, they are probably designed as much for playing around with the computer as for anything else. CompuServe has a number of clubs for professionals where ideas and even programs may be exchanged. It is still too early to assess how useful CompuServe customers find this type of service, as there is a dearth of research in the area. Apparently CompuServe has found that certain data bases generate interest. Whether that interest is recreational or a legitimate business interest is not yet known.

READABLE DATA BASES

Serious Data Bases

Computer Readable Data Bases lists over 100 medically oriented data bases, from *Abstracts on Health Effects of Environmental Pollutants* to the *Veterinary Bulletin*. These data bases provide up-to-date information regarding statistics and developments in their respective fields. Some also provide interactive services that assist the practitioner in arriving at a diagnosis.

Time and Charges

One of the biggest problems with most data bases is that the meter is running while you are using them. You might think differently about using a stereo if you were billed for each minute of use. It's not that data base management systems are inequitable, as in some respects they are the epitome of equity. One pays only for what one uses. It's not difficult to spend $1,200 or more for a 20-volume, hardbound encyclopedia, 80 percent of whose pages will never be accessed. With a computer data base, one establishes the parameters and within a few minutes the computer searches through several years of articles. A similar physical search at a library might take days. However, the total bill for the computer services might be only $10 or $15.

Efficiency

The byword of data base systems is efficiency. However, a data base system can be no more efficient than the user. Unfortunately, every system has its own series of commands and prompts. A dentist gives the following account:

> I don't consider myself an ignorant person, but it took me nearly two days of intermittent trying to access CompuServe, which I finally did, quite by accident. In none of the material I had available was there the simple statement "Press the Break key after accessing the Host." Terribly grateful to be logged on, I thought I would casually use the one hour of free service that was provided with my Videotex software package.
>
> In my preliminary reading I had fortunately learned that it's a good idea to turn the printer on before accessing CompuServe. This gives you a good hard copy of page references that flash across the screen. I soon found, however, that I appeared to be locked into an interminable program. My only choice was to "Press Enter to see next screen." Short of unplugging the computer or hitting reset, I was determined to find the answer to this problem. I quickly looked to the manual while I periodically "Pressed Enter to see next screen." I never did solve the problem. Eventually, about 10 minutes later, the program reached its logical conclusion and I was able to shift back to the main menu.

This situation emphasizes the problems entailed in learning the system. Although you pay only for the information you receive, in essence you also pay for learning how to use the system. Unless and until you learn how to move around in a data base, it can be a slow, sluggish, frustrating, and costly experience. It is not difficult to spend an hour a day with a data base. Even at the non-prime-time rate of $5 an hour, it is easy to see how this can add $1,200 a year to one's overhead. But what about prime-time rates of $72-plus an hour?

The Future

Electronic data bases are in their infancy. At the time this book was being written, the Dow Jones Free Text Search was available only during limited hours, but it was expected to soon be made available on weekends. CompuServe did not have any dental software packages, although it had a heading for them in the data base. Each month new telephone numbers are being provided in major cities giving access to many new data bases. It is clear that growth is expected.

For the practitioner who is willing to make the financial commitment, excellent systems are available to assist him in keeping abreast of up-to-the-minute developments in diagnosis and treatment. For the practitioner who wishes to dabble, a $150 modem and a $40 Videotex package (with Universal DJ/N and CompuServe sign-up kit) will bring him into the world of the 21st century.

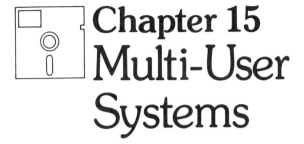

Chapter 15
Multi-User Systems

PICTURE THIS
RAMIFICATIONS
ADVANTAGES
    Speed
    Multiple Access
    Automatic Functions
    Software Savings
    Hardware Savings
DISADVANTAGES
    Cost
    Speed
    Confidentiality
THE FUTURE

PICTURE THIS

Picture this: It is 11 A.M. You are sitting in your office in front of your VDT. You have accessed CompuServe (see previous chapter) and have entered a code that will bring you in contact with a special interest group (SIG) that meets every Thursday morning to "discuss private practice management." This morning a practitioner from Denver will be presenting a paper on "New Developments in Malpractice Liability."

    In an adjacent office your associate has turned on her VDT to look over the charts of patients who have not been to the office in over a month. She will check disposition and determine whether or not a proper termination note has been entered. If she so desires, she may type in the information while she examines the charts.

Down the hall, in a smaller room, a patient is sitting in front of a VDT answering prompts to complete a medical history. It will be finished in a few minutes, and the patient will then take the MMPI by computer.

In the business office the secretary is involved in word processing. This morning she is collating clinical reports on patients produced by the doctors and the computer. A few yards from her, the bookkeeper is sorting out insurance forms that have just been printed on her dot matrix printer. While the bookkeeper is doing this, her VDT reads, "General ledger is being posted."

A few yards from the secretary and the bookkeeper is the CPU. It is as large as a three-drawer, legal-sized filing cabinet. At this moment a small green light is lit on the control panel. This means that one of the remote units is being used. In this case, it is a remote unit placed in a satellite office situated across town. There the MMPI is being administered to a patient. That information will be interpreted in a few minutes and become part of a report that will go out to the referring doctor.

RAMIFICATIONS

The above configuration might be considered by some to be the ideal computerized office. It permits multiple access from multiple locations to similar or disparate programs on a single powerful CPU. Provided by a consulting firm, this configuration will cost the practitioner between $50,000 and $75,000.

Multi-user systems require large memory (250K–900K bytes of RAM) and large storage capacities (12M–50M bytes). They also use 16-bit microprocessors, very sophisticated programs, and, of course, a multi-user operating system. It's probably feasible for the practitioner to put together a three-terminal system herself. All of the problems with single-user systems, discussed in earlier chapters, will increase, at least arithmetically (and perhaps geometrically), with multi-user systems. It's bad enough to have one person scratching her head in front of a VDT, but it's far worse if eight people have problems with the computer. Therefore, consultant relationships are more critical with more complicated systems. Below are listed the major advantages and disadvantages of a multi-user system.

ADVANTAGES

Speed

Because of its 16-bit operating system, a multi-user system, when not pressed by many users, performs more quickly than does its 8-bit single-user counterpart.

Multiple Access

This advantage is obvious. A multi-user computer may be given over to many operations at a given moment. At any one time, the secretary may be doing word processing, the bookkeeper may be posting a ledger, a practitioner may be checking on patient status, and a patient may be interacting with a VDT, providing information or taking tests.

Automatic Functions

Although a single-user system can be used with remote terminals, this is done more commonly with multi-user systems. Offices may be interconnected; information may be gleaned or retrieved overnight; and the system may be updated by a remote consultant.

Software Savings

Typically, software packages are licensed to be used on only one computer. Most software companies demand that the practitioner purchase, for example, a word processing program for every system on which it will be used. From the point of view of software investment, the multi-user systems are more economical, as only one software package is used for one CPU. It is neither necessary nor possible to buy a separate package for each CRT involved.

Hardware Savings

A multi-user system eliminates redundancy in the purchase of certain hardware components, the most noticeable of which is a CPU. In a multi-user system, one CPU services every CRT and printer, and for that matter every other output device.

DISADVANTAGES

For each advantage of the multi-user system, there is a contrasting disadvantage.

Cost

In the final analysis, a multi-user system may be more cost efficient than a single-user system, but the initial outlay is substantially higher. The guts of the operation are likely to cost about 30–50 percent more. In addition, more CRTs and cables, more sophisticated software and services, and more consultation services will be required.

Speed

Most multi-user systems will slow down as more operators use them. An individual may find herself closed out of a file because it is being accessed by someone else, or the general responsiveness of the system may slow to a grind as several users tax the memory of the CPU.

Confidentiality

Because a multi-user system is likely to be operable 24 hours a day and to be accessible by telephone and by a number of users, there is a greater risk of tampering. Although better safeguards are constantly being developed, it is fair to say that few systems will be able to survive a concentrated effort by a well-versed person who wishes to enter it. The improved safeguards will involve better password protection, that is, systems that shut down when tampered with or systems that monitor tampering and alert officials or owners.

THE FUTURE

Multi-user systems, like single-user systems, are being simplifed and reduced in price. At present, a number of major companies are releasing small-configuration multi-user systems. Software applicable to private practice management is quickly being developed for these systems. These developments will enable the practitioner to implement a multi-user system at reduced cost and with minimal external consultation.

Glossary*

address 1. A character or group of characters that identifies a register, a particular part of storage, or some other data source or destination. 2. To refer to a device or an item of data by its address.

applications program A program written to accomplish a specific user task (such as payroll) as opposed to supervisory, general-purpose, or utility programs.

BASIC Beginner's All-purpose Symbolic Instruction Code. A common high-level time-sharing computer programming language. It is easily learned. The language was developed by Dartmouth College.

baud 1. A unit of signaling speed equal to the number of discrete conditions or signal events per second. For example, one baud equals one-half dot cycle per second in Morse Code, one bit per second in a train of binary signals, and one 3-bit value per second in a train of signals, each of which can assume one of eight different states. 2. In asynchronous transmission, the unit of modulation rate corresponding to one unit interval per second, i.e., if the duration of the units interval is 20 milliseconds, the modulation rate is 50 baud.

baud rate A type of measurement of data flow in which the number of signal elements per second is based on the duration of the shortest element. When each element carries one bit, the baud rate is numerically equal to bits per second (bps).

benchmark In relation to microprocessors, the benchmark is a test point measuring the performance characteristics of products offered. A benchmark program is a routine or program selected to define or compare different brands of microprocessors. A flowchart in assembly language is often written out for each microprocessor, and the execution of the benchmark time, accuracy, etc., is evaluated.

bit Bit is an abbreviation for binary digit. Most commonly, a unit of information equaling one binary decision, or the designation of one of two possible and equally likely values or states. It is usually conveyed as a 1 or 0 of anything that can be used to store or convey information (such as 1 or 0, which may also mean "yes" or "no"). 2. A single character in a binary number. 3. A single pulse in a group of pulses. 4. A unit of information capacity of a storage device. The capacity in bits is the logarithm to the base two of the number of possible states of the device.

---

* The above definitions appear in Charles J. Sippl, *Microcomputer Dictionary*, Indianapolis: Howard W. Sams, Co., Inc., 1981, and are reprinted with permission of the publisher.

bootstrap A technique or device designed to bring itself into a desired state by means of its own action, e.g., a machine routine whose first few instructions are sufficient to bring the rest of the routine into the computer from an input device.

bubble memories These memories are actually tiny cylinders of magnetization whose axes lie perpendicular to the plane of the single-crystal sheet that contains them. Magnetic bubbles arise when two magnetic fields are applied perpendicular to the sheet. A constant field strengthens and fattens the regions of the sheet whose magnetization lies along it. A pulsed field then breaks the strengthened regions into isolated bubbles, which are free to move within the plane of the sheet. Because the presence or absence of bubbles can represent digital information and because other external fields can manipulate this information, magnetic bubble devices could find uses in future data-storage systems. However, the magnetic bubble memory needs various circuits to operate as a complete bubble memory system. These circuits include a controller (to provide a CPU interface and generate enable pulses to a function timing generator), coil and function drivers, and a sense amplifier (to amplify the signal of the bubble detector).

bug 1. A program defect or error. Also refers to any circuit fault due to improper design or construction. 2. A mistake or malfunction.

bus As applied to computer technology, one or more conductors used as a path over which information is transmitted.

byte A term used to indicate a specific number of consecutive bits often considered to consist of 8 bits which, as a unit, can represent one character or two numerals.

card cage 1. A unit designed to permit installation of pc cards (*see* 2. Card) without the necessity of hard-wiring. The card cages themselves are sturdy steel construction and usually include a retaining bar to ensure that cards cannot be shaken from their sockets. The cage backplanes include full sets of edge connectors soldered in place on the cage's bus. 2. Many suppliers offer one 12-connector card cage with a basic microprocessor. It is often prewired to hold the CPU, two memory cards, a front panel interface, and a card reader controller. An additional 6-connector card cage may be installed to allow for expansion. Generally, if still more expansion is required, the power supplies may be removed and installed remotely, thus providing space for an additional pair of 6-connector card cages (in some systems).

central processing unit (CPU) 1. A unit of a microcomputer that includes the circuits controlling the interpretation and execution of instructions. Synonymous with mainframe. 2. The central processor of a computer system contains main storage, arithmetic unit, control registers, and scratchpad memory.

chip 1. An unpackaged semiconductor device. A die from a silicon wafer incorporating an integrated circuit. 2. A tiny piece of semiconductor material on which microscopic electronic components are photoetched to form one or more circuits. After connection leads and a case are added to the chip, it is called an integrated circuit.

COBOL   Abbreviation for Common Business Oriented Language. 1. A data processing language that makes use of English language statements. 2. Pertaining to a computer program which translates a COBOL language program into a machine language program.

CP/M operating system   CP/M is the abbreviation for Control Program for Microprocessors. It is the registered trademark of Digital Research.

CRT   Abbreviation for cathode ray tube.

data base management   Refers to a software product that controls a data structure containing interrelated data stored so as to optimize accessibility, control redundancy, and provide or offer multiple views of the data to multiple applications programs.

disk crash   This refers to a disk Read/Write head making destructive contact with the surface of a rotating disk. Loosely refers to any disk unit failure that results in a system malfunction.

disk drives   Typical disk drives are highly reliable, random access, moving-head memory devices, compactly designed for use as peripheral units in large, small, and, now, microcomputer systems.

disk operating system (DOS)   Many such programs are data communications-oriented disk-based operating systems. They feature both multiterminal and multitasking capabilities and allow full control of both hardware and software operations through the system console, or any batch input device.

disk operating system, MP/M   MP/M is a popular small computer disk operating system that provides multiterminal access with multiprogramming at each terminal. It is compatible with its predecessor CP/M and, thus, can run many programming languages, applications packages, and development software created for various systems. It offers such advanced capabilities as run editors, translators, word processors, and background print spoolers. Users can write their own system processes for operation under MP/M.

documentation   Refers to the orderly presentation, organization, and communication of recorded specialized knowledge, in order to maintain a complete record of reasons for changes in variables. Documentation is necessary, not so much to give maximum utility, as to give an unquestionable historical reference record. Such documents usually contain: (1) The name of the responsible individual who ordered or is directing the program, (2) A brief outline of the system, with some notes relating to the benefits to be obtained, and (3) A type of "handbook" that is developed for use by those who will use the system and programs. It explains such things as paper flow, the coding required, and the output file instructions. Other items explained are equipment utilization change-over procedures, systems test data, program descriptions, etc.

floppy-disk systems A typical floppy disk provides random access program/data storage. Hard-sector formatted, each disk will hold over 300,000 data bytes.

glitch 1. An unwanted false electronic pulse. 2. Any of a variety of problems that can plague both hardware and software in digital designs.

hardware Refers to the metallic, or "hard" components of a microcomputer system in contrast to the "soft," or programming, components. The components of circuits may be active, passive, or both.

language A defined set of characters used to form symbols, words, etc., and the rules for combining these characters into meaningful communications, e.g., FORTRAN, C, COBOL, ALGOL, English, or French.

main frame The central processor of the computer system. It contains the main storage, arithmetic unit, and special register groups. (Synonymous with CPU and central processing unit.)

memory One of the three basic components of a CPU, memory stores information for future use. Storage and memory are interchangeable expressions. Memories accept and hold binary numbers or images.

modem Refers to a MODulation/DEModulation chip, or device, that enables computers and terminals to communicate over telephone circuits. A modulator/demodulator connects the communications multiplexer from the remote outlet to the interface device in the computer center.

MUMPS A text-oriented language with built-in data base facilities and string and pattern matching. Used in hospitals and other large organizations for unified accounting. The basic orientation of MUMPS is procedural, much like FORTRAN or COBOL. However, because of the interactive nature of the system, programs are written and fully debugged in a fraction of the time required by other high-level languages.

packaged software Also called "canned," it usually consists of generalized programs that are prewritten and debugged and are designed to perform one or more general business functions, such as accounts receivable, accounts payable, general ledger, payroll, or inventory control.

patch To correct or change the coding at a particular location by inserting transfer instructions at that location and by adding the new instructions and the replaced instructions elsewhere.

program 1. A set of instructions arranged in a proper sequence for directing a digital computer in performing a desired operation or operations (e.g., the solution of a mathematical problem or the collation of a set of data). 2. To prepare a program (as contrasted with "to code").

RAM Abbreviation for random access memory. This type memory is random because it provides immediate access to any storage location point in the memory by means of vertical and horizontal coordinates. Information may be "written in" or "read out" in the same very fast procedure.

read To copy, usually from one form of storage to another, particularly from external or secondary storage to internal storage.

ROM Abbreviation for read-only memory device where information is store permanently or semipermanently and can be read out but not altered in operation.

ROM bootstrap Nearly every computer uses at least one ROM program, the most common one being a ROM bootstrap loader. The bootstrap loader is a minimum program which, if everything in memory has been wiped out, will allow the programmer to recreate the main memory load.

RS-232 interface Refers to the interface between a modem and the associated data-terminal equipment.

software 1. The term *software* was invented to contrast with the "iron" or hardware, of a computer system. Software items are programs, languages, and procedures of a computer system. Software libraries for microprocessors are being built and assembled with heavy competition among suppliers, both manufacturers and distributors. 2. Refers to the internal programs or routines prepared professionally to simplify programming and computer operations. Uses permit the programmer to use his own language (English) or mathematics (algebra) in communicating with the computer. 3. The various programming aids that are frequently supplied by the manufacturers to facilitate the purchaser's efficient operation of the equipment. Such software items include various assemblers, generators, subroutine libraries, compilers, operating systems, and industry-application programs.

spooling Refers to a procedure of temporarily storing data on disk or tape files until another aspect of processing is ready for the data (such as printing it).

transient The instantaneous surge of voltage or current, produced by a change from one steady-state condition to another.

turnkey A design and/or installation in which the user receives a complete running system.

utilities A group of programs performing duties, such as program check-out, editing, word processing, text preparation, and accounting, that are standard software or installation implemented. Used on all systems.

References

Bayer, B. D., and J. J. Sobel. *Dynamics of VisiCalc ®*. Homewood, Ill.: Dow Jones-Irwin, 1983.

Brinbaum, M., and J. Sickman. *How to Choose a Business Computer*. Reading, Mass.: Addison-Wesley Publishing, 1982.

Canning, R. G., and N. C. Leeper. *So You Are Thinking about a Small Business Computer: 1982–83 Edition*. Englewood Cliffs, N.J.: Prentice-Hall, 1982.

Covvey, H. D., and N. H. McAllister. *Computer Consciousness: Surviving the Automated 80s*. Reading, Mass.: Addison-Wesley Publishing, 1980.

Deken, J. *The Electronic Cottage: Everyday Living with Your Personal Computer in the 1980s*. New York: William Morrow, 1981.

Dow Jones News/Retrieval Fact Finder. New York: Dow Jones News/Retrieval, 1983.

Fluegelman, A., and J. J. Hewes. *Writing in the Computer Age: Word Processing Skills and Style for Every Writer*. Garden City, N.Y.: Anchor Books, 1983.

Frude, Neil. "The Affectionate Machine." *Psychology Today,* December 1983, pp. 23–24.

Glossbrenner, A. *The Complete Handbook of Personal Computer Communications: Everything You Need to Go Online with the World*. New York: St. Martin's Press, 1983.

Greenwood, Frank. *Profitable Small Business Computing: Practical Guide to Finding and Using the Right Computer for Your Business Needs*. Boston: Little, Brown, 1982.

Herbert, F. *Without Me, You're Nothing: The Essential Guide to Home Computers*. New York: Pocket Books, 1982.

Holitzman, C. P. *What to Do When You Get Your Hands on a Microcomputer*. Blue Ridge Summit, PA: Tab Books.

Kitter, T. *The Soul of a New Machine*. New York: Avon Books, 1981.

Klein, Judy Graf. *The Office Book*. New York: Facts on File, 1982.

Levy, S. "Modem Wars." *Popular Computing,* August 1983, p. 71.

McWilliams, Peter A. *The Word Processing Book: A Short Course in Computer Literacy*. Los Angeles: Prelude Press, 1982.

————. *The Personal Computer Book*. Los Angeles: Prelude Press, 1982.

———. *The Personal Computer in Business Book.* Los Angeles: Prelude Press, 1983.

Nims, F., and editors of Consumer's Guide. *Easy to Understand Guide to Home Computers.* Publications International Limited, 1982.

Pressman, Robert M. *Private Practice: A Handbook for the Independent Mental Health Practitioner.* New York: Gardner Press, 1979.

Pressman, Robert M., and Rodie Siegler. *The Independent Practitioner: Practice Management for the Allied Health Professional.* Homewood, Ill.: Dow Jones-Irwin, 1983.

"Product Highlight." *Interface Age,* August 1983, p. 16.

Schwartz, Marc D., M.D. *Using Computers in Clinical Practice: Psychotherapy and Mental Health Applications.* New York: Haworth Press, 1983.

Shaw, D. R. *Small Business Computer: Evaluating, Selecting, Financing, Installing and Operating the Hardware and Software that Fits.* Parsippany, N.J.: Business Counselors, 1981.

Sippl, Charles J. *Microcomputer Dictionary.* Indianapolis, Ind.: Howard W. Sams, 1981.

Slesin, L., and Martha Zybko. Video Display Terminals: Health and Safety. Excerpts from *Microwave News,* New York, 1983.

Stair, Ralph M., Jr. *Learning to Live with Computers: Advice for Managers.* Homewood, Ill.: Dow Jones-Irwin, 1983.

Stollard, J. J.; E. R. Smith; and D. Reese. *The Electronic Office: A Guide for Managers.* Homewood, Ill.: Dow Jones-Irwin, 1983.

Tandy Corporation and Management Consultants for Professionals. *Medical Office System Program Manual,* 1983.

Walker, R. *Understanding Computer Science.* Texas Instruments, 1981.

Walter, R. *The Secret Guide to Computers.* Boston: Russ Walter.

Zaks, R. *Don't: Or How to Care for Your Computer.* SYBEX, 1981.

Annotated Bibliography

Bayer, B. D. and J. J. Sobel. *Dynamics of VisiCalc®*. Homewood, Ill.: Dow Jones-Irwin, 1983. $19.95

This is the first guide for business users of VisiCalc, the best-selling microcomputer program, which has become the businessperson's partner in revising budgets; writing business plans; projecting profits, sales, and trends; and more. Any manager who wants to develop sophisticated applications using VisiCalc or merely understand the program will benefit from this practical guide.

Brinbaum, M., and J. Sickman. *How to Choose a Business Computer*. Reading, Mass.: Addison-Wesley Publishing, 1982.

A book laid out well with helpful charts and diagrams. Two major sections on what the computer market offers and how to computerize your business provide outstanding guides.

Canning, R. G., and N. C. Leeper. *So You Are Thinking about a Small Business Computer: 1982–1983 Edition*. Englewood Cliffs, N.J.: Prentice-Hall, 1982.

Forms and questionnaires are included to help analyze computer needs, i.e., estimates of average data entry workload, printer wordload, computer capacity, etc. The text is organized in a broad, double-column quality paperback, which is easy to read. It is replete with information to assist the businessmen and women in choosing the right equipment.

Covvey, H. D., and N. H. McAllister. *Computer Consciousness: Surviving the Automated 80s*. Reading, Mass.: Addison-Wesley Publishing, 1980.

Another successful, lightly written book designed for the novice. Illustrations and flowcharts are well done and provide the reader with a good working knowledge of computer software, hardware, and communications technology. A commonsense pricing guide is also provided.

Deken, J. *The Electronic Cottage: Everyday Living with Your Personal Computer in the 1980s*. New York: William Morrow, 1981.

Now in paperback; however, this classic is worth the investment in the hardcover version. Even if you never purchase or use a computer, the book is worth reading for its excellent prose. The author probably could successfully teach computer science to an entire geriatric ward. He has a gift for imaginative and helpful verbal illustrations. But moreover, he lifts the reader from the confusing electronic world of today into the exciting and understandable world which may yet come to be.

Fluegelman, A., and J. J. Hewes. *Writing in the Computer Age: Word Processing Skills and Style for Every Writer.* Garden City, N.Y.: Anchor Books, 1983.

This book is packed with practical ways of getting the most out of any word processing system. Advice is given regarding writing styles and strategies, editing and polishing manuscripts, as well as organizing information and participating in networking programs. This book is highly recommended for anyone seriously involved in word processing.

Glossbrenner, A. *The Complete Handbook of Personal Computer Communications: Everything You Need to Go Online with the World.* New York: St. Martin's Press, 1983. $14.95.

This book is a must for anyone involved in telecomputing. The cost of the book will soon be recouped by learning how to use CompuServe, The Source, and Dow Jones News Retrieval Service with greater efficiency. There are also sections on computer banking, shopping, mail, and typesetting. Common problems and methods of getting around them are discussed.

Greenwood, Frank. *Profitable Small Business Computing: Practical Guide to Finding and Using the Right Computer for Your Business Needs.* Boston: Little, Brown, 1982.

A practical guide for getting maximum use from microcomputers. About three fifths of the book is devoted to finding the most appropriate equipment; the remaining two fifths, for getting maximal use of the equipment and software once you acquire it.

Herbert, F. *Without Me, You're Nothing: The Essential Guide to Home Computers.* New York: Pocket Books, 1982.

Somewhat of a hyperbole by title, the book nevertheless is complete. There is an attempt to provide both substance and humor (as is the current trend in writing about computers). Two useful chapters are "What's Your Name, Funny Machine?" and "History Without Hysteria."

Holitzman, C. P. *What to Do When You Get Your Hands on a Microcomputer.* Blue Ridge Summit, Pa: Tab Books, hardbound $16.95.

One of the more painless how-to-do-it books on BASIC. The volume is nicely laid out and has lots of white space and illustrations. The doctor or teenage reader will walk away from this book with a working knowledge of BASIC commands.

Kitter, T. *The Soul of a New Machine.* New York: Avon Books, 1981.

This best-selling fiction and 1982 Pulitzer Prize winner will give the reader some idea of the intrigue that goes on in the development of popular computers.

McWilliams trilogy. This is not a book but rather three popular and informative quality paperbacks written by Peter A. McWilliams. They are *The Word Processing Book: A Short Course in Computer Literacy,* 1982; *The Personal Computer Book,* 1982; and *The Personal Computer in Business Book,* 1983.

All are published by Prelude Press in Los Angeles and cost about $10. In the introduction of the latter, William F. Buckley, Jr., states, "The author of this book was born to write pleasantly about subjects one is instinctively fearful of. If we go back to capital punishment in a big way, I shall suggest McWilliams be given the job of writing the manual on how to operate electric chairs so as not to run the risk of getting hurt." Each is written with a unique combination of humor and on-the-target information. The reader will walk away with a few belly laughs plus insights. *The Word Processing Book* and *The Personal Computer Book* are good volumes to have while agonizing about whether to buy a computer. *The Personal Computer in Business Book* is nice to have while you are agonizing after buying a computer.

Nims, F., and editors of Consumer's Guide. *Easy to Understand Guide to Home Computers.* Publications International Limited, 1982.

In the world of computers, this is an inexpensive paperback ($3.95). It's the type of publication that you might carry on to an airplane or elsewhere to leaf through. It contains a number of helpful features, including illustrations, photographs, glossary, and a short buying guide. It also has an excellent index.

Schwartz, Marc D., M.D. *Using Computers in Clinical Practice: Psychotherapy and Mental Health Applications.* New York: Haworth Press, 1983.

This up-to-date volume provides massive detail about computer use in the clinical practice of psychology. The short and plentiful chapters give the practitioner a good taste of the many uses, problems, and solutions that computers offer a psychologist.

Shaw, D. R. *Small Business Computer: Evaluating, Selecting, Financing, Installing and Operating the Hardware and Software that Fits.* Parsippany, N.J.: Business Counselors, 1981.

The title speaks for itself. The strength of this book lies in helping the practitioner deal effectively with computer vendors. It is geared more toward larger businesses than private practices. Nonetheless, it has practical advice regarding requests for proposals, negotiating a contract and implementing a computer system.

Stair, Ralph M., Jr. *Learning to Live With Computers: Advice for Managers.* Homewood, Ill.: Dow Jones-Irwin, 1983. $19.95.

This volume clearly and precisely explains how to put a computer to maximum use while avoiding common pitfalls. It covers: the state of the art in hardware, software, and peripheral equipment; how to acquire software and hardware; how to combine hardware and software into an effective system; and the sources and suppliers in the computer industry. The necessary steps to either purchase or develop your own software are also included.

Stallard, J. J.; E. R. Smith; and D. Reese. *The Electronic Office: A Guide for Managers.* Homewood, Ill.: Dow Jones-Irwin, 1983. $19.95.

In these guidelines, designing, acquiring, and managing an integrated office automation system, the authors fully explain the use of a word processor. They also show how it is related to dictation equipment and to reprographic and micrographic equipment as well as how it contributes to efficient management and retrieval of documents. Checklists and questionnaires give managers the extra edge they need to ensure a smooth transition from traditional office to automated procedures.

Walker, R. *Understanding Computer Science.* Texas Instruments, 1981.

Although dry, this book has a thorough format and could be used as the text in a college course Computer Science 101. It is complete with quizzes at the end of each chapter to provide readers with an opportunity to judge their own progress. It is distributed in paperback and offered at Radio Shack stores.

Walter, R. *The Secret Guide to Computers.* A self-published series of books by Russ Walter, 92 St. Botolph, Boston, MA 02116.

At $3.70 each, these paperbacks are possibly one of the cheapest and most informative sources in the computer book market.

Zaks, R. *Don't: Or How to Care for Your Computer.* SYBEX, 1981.

> Practically every conceivable problem that might occur in using a computer is listed in this book. There are, of course, suggestions for avoiding these problems. It is replete with illustrations, cartoons, and photographs to provide humor and impact. One cartoon shows a man engrossed in reading his newspaper and ignoring his paper-jammed computer, which is producing flames about one foot high. The book will go a long way in helping the practitioner keep out of trouble and to understand about the practical side and intricacies of computer technology.

Appendix A

Examples of Computer Reports on Practice Activity*

1. Day Sheet Summary, Part 1
2. Day Sheet Summary, Part 2
3. Day Sheet Summary, Part 3
4. Production Report
5. Open Contracts Report
6. Management Survey
7. Production Analysis

---

*Reprinted by permission of Safeguard Business Systems, Inc., Fort Washington, Pennsylvania 19034.

1. Day Sheet Summary, Part 1

This report gives a detailed recap of all procedures and transactions which transpire during the day. Information is entered from typical pegboard system.

```
6/01/83  10:13 AM                                    MEDICAL DEMONSTRATION                                              Page    1
Doc 1: JOHN J JONES MD                                 DAY SHEET SUMMARY                                               NUMBER   6

FAMILY   PAT    STAFF  TRANS     PATIENT    FIRST    M                                    EST    ADJ      C            C    ADJ
  ID     ID    PRI DR  DATE     LAST NAME   NAME     I  PROC   DESCRIPTION       LOC CHARGE    INS  CHARGE    D PAYMENT    D CREDIT

ABBOT    THOMA    1    6/01/83  ABBOT       THOMAS   T. 90620  CONSULTATION C      O  100.00   0.00   0.00
ACE      FRANC    3    6/01/83  ACE         FRANCES     90220  HOSPITAL VISIT     IH   50.00   0.00                BS*  14.12  CD*   3.11
BENNETT  RICHA    1    6/01/83  BENNETT     RICHARD     90040  OFFICE VISIT  C    IH   45.00   0.00                BS    25.00
BROWN2   MARY     1    6/01/83  BROWN       MARY     J. 90040  OFFICE VISIT  C     O   45.00   0.00                CK    35.00
BROWN3   JOHN     1    6/01/83  BROWN       JOHN     J.                                                            BS*    4.08
CABOT    JOHN     3    6/01/83  CABOT       JOHN     J. 90620  CONSULTATION C      O  100.00   0.00                TR    35.00  IA    7.00
CARD     JAMES    1    6/01/83  CARD        JAMES       90020  OFFICE VISIT  I    IH   30.00   0.00
CASS     JAMES    1    6/01/83  CASS        JAMES
CLUB     PATRI    1    6/01/83  CLUB        PATRICK     90040  OFFICE VISIT  C     H   45.00   0.00                CA    48.68
CLUB     PATRI    1    6/01/83  CLUB        PATRICK     I 1    UA-LAB CHARGE      IL   12.00   0.00
HEART    MARY     1    6/01/83  HEART       MARY        I 1    UA-LAB CHARGE      IL   12.00   0.00                PR*  114.35
HEART    MARY     1    6/01/83  HEART       MARY        I 2    CHOLER.-LAB CH     IL   12.00   0.00
HEART    MARY     1    6/01/83  HEART       MARY        I 3    CREAT.BLD.LAB      IL   12.00   0.00
HEART    MARY     1    6/01/83  HEART       MARY        I 4    FBS LAB CHARGE     IL   12.00   0.00                CA*    8.11
PARKER   JOHN     1    6/01/83  PARKER      JOHN        90030  OFFICE VISIT  E     O   30.00   0.00                CK*    6.99  IA*   1.60
QUEEN    KATHL    3    6/01/83  QUEEN       KATHLEEN

DOCTOR TOTALS:             DAY SHEET:                                                505.00   0.00   0.00             291.33       11.71

                           MONTH TO DATE:                                           1394.68 137.20   0.00             886.89       18.52

                           FISCAL YTD:                                              2076.68 137.20   0.00            1065.31       56.02

                           CURRENT ACCOUNTS RECEIVABLE      955.35                                     * DENOTES ALLOCATION
```

2. Day Sheet Summary, Part 2

This report redistributes information from the day sheet so that each doctor in a group practice may analyze the daily composite of those patients seen and charges/payments recorded.

```
6/01/83  10:13 AM                          MEDICAL DEMONSTRATION                                                    Page  2
                                             DAY SHEET SUMMARY                                                     NUMBER  6
Doc 1: JOHN J JONES MD

FAMILY  PAT  STAFF  TRANS  PATIENT   FIRST  M                                    EST      ADJ      C          C    ADJ
  ID    ID   PRI DR  DATE  LAST NAME  NAME  I  PROC  DESCRIPTION  LOC  CHARGE    INS    CHARGE   D PAYMENT    D  CREDIT

CHARGES AND CHARGE ADJUSTMENTS ON:        ------ MY PATIENTS ------        -- OTHER DOCTOR'S PATIENTS --
DOCTOR                                DAILY      MONTH TO DATE             DAILY       MONTH TO DATE
NO. NAME                              AMOUNT        AMOUNT                 AMOUNT         AMOUNT
 1  JOHN J JONES MD                   455.00       1169.68
 2  STEVEN A BLACK MD                  30.00        212.00
 3  LINDA L. LAUDER, M.D.                                                   50.00         225.00

STAFF WORK FOR ME
STAFF                                 DAILY      MONTH TO DATE
NO. NAME                              AMOUNT        AMOUNT

PAYMENTS ALLOCATED FROM:                  ------ MY FAMILIES ------        -- OTHER DOCTOR'S FAMILIES --
DOCTOR                                DAILY      MONTH TO DATE             DAILY       MONTH TO DATE
NO. NAME                              AMOUNT        AMOUNT                 AMOUNT         AMOUNT
 1  JOHN J JONES MD                   266.14        726.51                  0.00          20.00
 2  STEVEN A BLACK MD                 112.54        284.67                 25.19         140.38
 3  LINDA L. LAUDER, M.D.               0.00         80.00

CREDIT ADJUSTMENTS ALLOCATED FROM:        ------ MY FAMILIES ------        -- OTHER DOCTOR'S FAMILIES --
DOCTOR                                DAILY      MONTH TO DATE             DAILY       MONTH TO DATE
NO. NAME                              AMOUNT        AMOUNT                 AMOUNT         AMOUNT
 1  JOHN J JONES MD                     7.00         10.33
 2  STEVEN A BLACK MD                   0.00          1.67
 3  LINDA L. LAUDER, M.D.                                                   4.71           8.19
```

3. Day Sheet Summary, Part 3

This report provides tabulations of charges and payments by day, month, and year.

```
6/01/83  10:13 AM                    MEDICAL DEMONSTRATION                                      Page   1
PRACTICE TOTALS                        DAY SHEET SUMMARY                                      NUMBER   6

FAMILY  PAT  STAFF  TRANS                                                    ADJ    C           C  ADJ
  ID     ID  PRI DR DATE  PATIENT    FIRST  M                       EST    CHARGE  D PAYMENT   D  CREDIT
                          LAST NAME  NAME   I  PROC  DESCRIPTION LOC CHARGE  INS

                    GRAND TOTALS:     DAY SHEET:              1345.00  121.00   0.00  1482.32    24.75

                                      MONTH TO DATE:          4764.25  572.74   0.00  3437.12    41.70

                                      FISCAL YTD:             7114.25  627.49   0.00  4190.12   121.70

                                      CURRENT ACCOUNTS RECEIVABLE   2802.43

                    BANK DEPOSIT TOTAL:  1482.32
                    CREDIT CARD TOTAL:      0.00
```

158

4. Production Report (by location)

This report is used by practices providing service at multiple locations. It provides details regarding charges and productivity at each location.

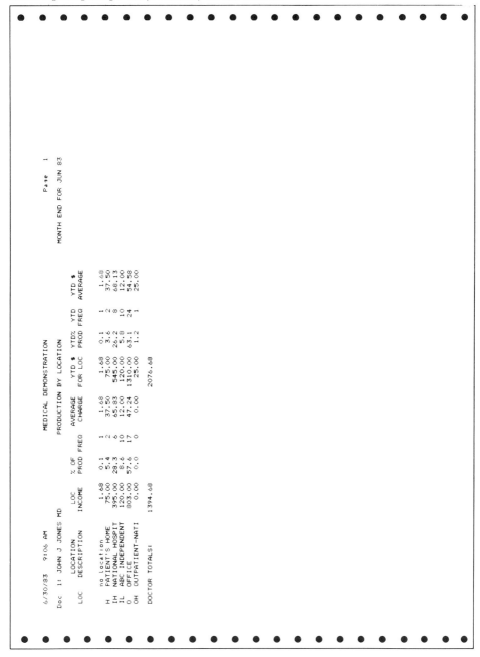

5. Open Contracts Report

This report provides details of financial contracts (installment payments) between patients and doctor.

```
6/01/83  12:06 PM                           MEDICAL DEMONSTRATION                                          Page  1

Doc  2: STEVEN A BLACK MD
                                                OPEN CONTRACTS

FAMILY  PATIENT                      CONTRACT           -INITIAL  PAYMENT-    FIRST    MONTHLY    ---REMAINING--
  ID      ID       NAME               NUMBER   CONTRACT   DATE     AMOUNT    PAYMENT   PAYMENT    PYMTS  BALANCE
                                               AMOUNT

SPORT   MAURE   MAUREEN SPORT            1      600.00  6/01/83   150.00     6/ 83      90.00       5     450.00
ZONE    BARRY   BARRY ZONE               1     1200.00  6/01/83   200.00     6/ 83     111.12       9    1000.00

DOCTORS TOTALS:                                1800.00                                 201.12            1450.00

SCHEDULED CHARGES BY MONTH 1-12:
JUN:  201.12   JUL:  201.12   AUG:  201.12   SEP:  201.12   OCT:  201.12   NOV:  111.12
DEC:  111.12   JAN:  111.12   FEB:  111.12   MAR:    0.00   APR:    0.00   MAY:    0.00
```

160

6. Management Survey

This report provides details regarding collections of accounts.

```
6/30/83   9:06 AM                          MEDICAL DEMONSTRATION
Doc  1: JOHN J JONES MD                 PRACTICE MANAGEMENT SUMMARY                            Page  1
                                                                                    MONTH END FOR JUN 83
                              PRESENT MO   PREVIOUS MO   3 MO AVERAGE    %       YEAR TO      %
                                 JUN          MAY        APR MAY JUN   CHANGE     DATE      CHANGE
-----MONTHLY TOTALS-----
BEGINNING ACCOUNTS RECEIVABLE    466.08        0.00         233.04       0.0        0.00      0.0

CHARGES                         1393.00      682.00        1037.50       0.0     2075.00      0.0
CHARGE ADJUSTMENTS                 0.00        0.00           0.00       0.0        0.00      0.0
FINANCE CHARGES                    1.68        0.00           0.84       0.0        1.68      0.0

PAYMENTS                         886.89CR    178.42CR       532.66CR     0.0     1065.31CR    0.0
CREDIT ADJUSTMENTS                18.52CR     37.50CR        28.01CR     0.0       56.02CR    0.0
SMALL BALANCE WRITE-OFF            0.00        0.00           0.00       0.0        0.00      0.0

ENDING ACCOUNTS RECEIVABLE       955.35      466.08         710.72       0.0      955.35      0.0

COLLECTION PERCENTAGE             63.7

--RECEIVABLES ANALYSIS--

RECEIVABLES AGING             PERCENTAGE

CREDIT BALANCES                   -0.6        6.00CR           0.00       0.0
CURRENT RECEIVABLES               95.0      908.03           529.02       0.0
OVER  30 DAYS                      0.0        0.00            64.54       0.0
OVER  60 DAYS                      0.0        0.00            93.50       0.0
OVER  90 DAYS                      6.6       63.32            31.66       0.0
OVER 120 DAYS                      0.0        0.00             0.00       0.0
ENDING BALANCE                   100.0      955.35           710.72       0.0

RECEIVABLES RATIO                  0.69       0.68            0.69       0.0

RECEIVABLES ON CONTRACT            0.0        0.00            0.00       0.0
RECEIVABLES CONTRACT NEXT MO.      0.0        0.00            0.00       0.0
RECEIVABLES ON INSURANCE          15.8      151.33           75.67       0.0
RECEIVABLES NOT BILLED             0.0        0.00            0.00       0.0

PAYMENT ON CURRENT CHARGES        50.9      486.65          215.92      351.29    44.4     0.0

-----ACTIVITY TOTALS-----

NEW PATIENTS ADDED                 2            9              6                  11       0.0
PATIENTS DELETED                   0            0              0                   0       0.0
PATIENTS ON FILE                  11            9             10                  11       0.0
FAMILIES ON FILE                  11            9             10                  11       0.0
STATEMENTS SENT                    7            0              4                   7       0.0
RECALLS SENT                       1            0              1                   1       0.0
RECALLS ENTERED                    0            4              2                   4       0.0

PERCENTAGE IN RECALL              45.5         44.4          50.0                 81.8     0.0
```

161

7. Production Analysis

This report analyzes various types of practice variables.

```
6/30/83  9:06 AM                          MEDICAL DEMONSTRATION                                          Page   1
Doc  1: JOHN J JONES MD                   PRODUCTION ANALYSIS                              MONTH END FOR JUN 83

  PROC    PROCEDURE                    MONTHLY  % OF   MO.  AVERAGE              %    YTD   AVERAGE
  CODE    DESCRIPTION                  PROD $   PROD  FREQ  CHARGE    $YTD      YTD  FREQ   CHARGE
                                                                    PROCEDURE

  81000   URINALYSIS                     36.00   2.6    3    12.00    48.00    2.3    4     12.00
  90020   OFFICE VISIT INTERMEDIATE      60.00   4.3    2    30.00    60.00    2.9    2     30.00
  90030   OFFICE VISIT EXTENDED          90.00   6.5    3    30.00    90.00    4.3    3     30.00
  90040   OFFICE VISIT COMPREHENSIVE    225.00  16.1    5    45.00   270.00   13.0    6     45.00
  90220   HOSPITAL VISIT COMPREHENSIVE  200.00  14.3    4    50.00   200.00    9.6    4     50.00
  90289   EMERGENCY ROOM                  0.00   0.0    0     0.00    25.00    1.2    1     25.00
  90600   CONSULTATION LTD                0.00   0.0    0     0.00   150.00    7.2    2     75.00
  90620   CONSULTATION COMPREHENSIVE    500.00  35.9    5   100.00   800.00   38.5    8    100.00
  93000   ECG COMP. WITH INTER/REPORT   150.00  10.8    2    75.00   300.00   14.4    4     75.00
  FINANCE FINANCE CHARGE                  1.68   0.1    1     1.68     1.68    0.1    1      1.68
  I 1     UA-LAB CHARGE $5.66            36.00   2.6    3    12.00    36.00    1.7    3     12.00
  I 2     CHOLER.-LAB CHARGE $5.66       24.00   1.7    2    12.00    24.00    1.2    2     12.00
  I 3     CREAT.BLD.LAB CHARGE $5.66     36.00   2.6    3    12.00    36.00    1.7    3     12.00
  I 4     FBS LAB CHARGE $5.66           24.00   1.7    2    12.00    24.00    1.2    2     12.00
  I 5     CBC LAB CHARGE $5.66           12.00   0.9    1    12.00    12.00    0.6    1     12.00

DOCTOR TOTALS:                         1394.68                       2076.68
```

Appendix B

Health Insurance Claim Form—HCFA 1500/CHAMPUS 501 (C-3)

Health Insurance Claim Form—HCFA 1500/CHAMPUS 501 (C-3)

Appendix C
Practice Analysis Utilizing Computer Graphics

1. All Transactions for One Month (December 1983)
2. Write-Offs for One Year (1983)

1. All Transactions for One Month (December 1983)

```
                    M O N T H   A T   A   G L A N C E

                          For Month 12  Year 1983

$7,964      .        00000        .                                       .
$7,466      .        00000        .                                       .
$6,969      .  00000 00000        .                                       .
$6,471      .  00000 00000        .                                       .
$5,973      .  00000 00000  00000 .                                       .
$5,475      .  00000 00000  00000 .                                       .
$4,977      .  00000 00000  00000 .                                       .
$4,480      .  00000 00000  00000 .                                       .
$3,982      .  00000 00000  00000 .                                       .
$3,484      .  00000 00000  00000 .                                       .
$2,986      .  00000 00000  00000 00000                                   .
$2,488      .  00000 00000  00000 00000                                   .
$1,991      .  00000 00000  00000 00000                                   .
$1,493      .  00000 00000  00000 00000                                   .
  $995      .  00000 00000  00000 00000  00000                            .
  $497      .  00000 00000  00000 00000  00000 00000 00000                .
   $0       .  00000 00000  00000 00000  00000 00000 00000 00000 00000 00000
            .........................................................
              Total  New    Pat   Ins    Adj P Adj I Adj   A/R   Cash  Write
              Recpt  Charg  Paym  Paym   Paym  Paym  Chrgs Due   In    Offs
```

2. All Write-Offs for One Year (1983)

```
                    Y E A R   A T   A   G L A N C E

                              Year 1983
                             $12,658.70
WRITE-OFFS
         ................................................................
  $3,190 .
  $2,991 .
  $2,791 .              00000
  $2,592 .              00000
  $2,392 .              00000                              00000
  $2,193 .              00000                              00000
  $1,994 .              00000                              00000
  $1,794 .              00000                              00000
  $1,595 .              0000000000                         00000
  $1,395 .              0000000000                         00000
  $1,196 .              000000000000            00000      00000
    $997 .    00000     000000000000            00000      00000
    $797 .    00000     000000000000            00000      00000
    $598 .    00000     000000000000            00000      00000
    $398 .    0000000000000000000000            000000000000000
    $199 .    0000000000000000000000000000000000000000000000000
      $0 .0000000000000000000000000000000000000000000000000000000000
         ................................................................
         Jan  Feb  Mar  Apr  May  Jun  Jul  Aug  Sep  Oct  Nov  Dec
```

Appendix D

Example of Computer Scored and Interpreted MMPI*

---
*Reprinted with permission of Interpretive Scoring Systems, a division of National Computer Systems

```
                            TM*
              THE MINNESOTA REPORT                    Page 1
                                        TM
for the Minnesota Multiphasic Personality Inventory  : Adult System

              By James N. Butcher, Ph.D.
```

Client No. : 27   Gender : Male
Setting : Mental Health Outpatient   Age :   34
Report Date : 14-FEB-84
ISS Code Number :   105 0002

PROFILE VALIDITY

   This is a valid MMPI profile. The client was quite cooperative in describing his symptoms and problems. His frank and open response to the items can be viewed as a positive indication of the individual's involvement with the evaluation. The MMPI profile is probably a good indication of his present personality functioning and symptoms.

SYMPTOMATIC PATTERN

   Individuals with this MMPI profile tend to show a pattern of chronic psychological maladjustment. The client appears to be quite anxious and depressed at this time. He may be feeling much somatic stress along with his psychological problems and may want relief from situational pressures.

   Apparently quite immature and hedonistic, he may act out impulsively and may show a recent history of acting-out behavior and substance abuse which resulted in considerable situational stress. He shows a pattern of superficial guilt or remorse over his behavior, but does not accept much responsibility for his actions. He may avoid confrontation and deny problems.

   He may experience some conflicts concerning his sex-role identity. He seems somewhat insecure in his masculine role, showing a generally feminine pattern of interests. He may be somewhat uncomfortable in relationships with women.

   His response content indicates that he is preoccupied with feeling guilty and unworthy, and feels that he deserves to be punished for wrongs he has committed. He feels regretful and unhappy about life, complains about having no zest for life, and seems plagued by anxiety and worry about the future. He has difficulty managing routine affairs, and the item content he endorsed suggests a poor memory, concentration problems, and an inability to make decisions. He appears to be immobilized and withdrawn and has no energy for life. According to his response content, there is a strong possibility that he has seriously contemplated suicide. A careful evaluation of this possibility is suggested.

NOTE: This MMPI interpretation can serve as a useful source of hypotheses about clients. This report is based on objectively derived scale indexes and scale interpretations that have been developed in diverse groups of patients. The personality descriptions, inferences and recommendations contained herein need to be verified by other sources of clinical information since individual clients may not fully match the prototype. The information in this report should most appropriately be used by a trained, qualified test interpreter. The information contained in this report should be considered confidential.

Client No. : 27   Report Date : 14-FEB-84   Page 2

INTERPERSONAL RELATIONS

He is probably experiencing disturbed interpersonal relationships, possibly owing to his acting-out behavior. While he appears to be socially outgoing, he relates to others superficially and may feel uncomfortable around others at this time.

BEHAVIORAL STABILITY

Individuals with this profile tend to have long-standing personality problems and are presently experiencing situational distress. Although they might express a desire to change, and feel remorseful over past behavior, they tend to change only temporarily, eventually drifting back into the old pattern.

DIAGNOSTIC CONSIDERATIONS

Individuals with this profile are often diagnosed as having a Personality Disorder (Dependent or Passive-Aggressive type) with a Substance Use Disorder.

TREATMENT CONSIDERATIONS

Individuals with this profile often show a "honeymoon" effect in therapy. They may verbalize a great need for help and show early gains, but as frustration mounts, they may fail treatment or terminate prematurely.

These individuals often are seeking a temporary haven from situational pressure. They are probably experiencing multiple problems which make it difficult to focus treatment. They are often predisposed to substance use and abuse disorders.

Any treatment program involving medications should be carefully evaluated. Since some individuals with this profile attempt to manipulate others through suicidal gestures, this possibility should also be taken into consideration.

MINNESOTA MULTIPHASIC PERSONALITY INVENTORY
Copyright THE UNIVERSITY OF MINNESOTA
1943, Renewed 1970. This Report 1982. All rights reserved.
Scored and Distributed Exclusively by NCS INTERPRETIVE SCORING SYSTEMS
Under License From The University of Minnesota

* "The Minnesota Report," "MMPI," and "Minnesota Multiphasic Personality Inventory" are trademarks owned by the University Press of the University of Minnesota.

THE MINNESOTA REPORT   Page 3
                    By James N. Butcher, Ph.D.

Client No. : 27   Gender : Male
Setting : Mental Health Outpatient   Age : 34
Report Date : 14-FEB-84

```
110- --------------- I ------------------------------------------ -110
  -                 I                                              -
  -                 I                                              -
  -                 I                                              -
  -                 I                                              -
100-                I                                              -100
  -                 I                                              -
  -                 I                                              -
  -                 I                                              -
  -                 I     *                                        -
 90-                I                                              -90
  -                 I                              *               -
  -                 I                                              -
  -                 I                                              -
  -                 I                                              -
 80-                I                                              -80
  -                 I                                              -
  -                 I          *                                   -
  -                 I                                              -
  -                 I                                *       *     -
 70- --------------- I -*-------------------*---------------------- -70
  -                 I                                              -
  -                 I       *           *                          -
  -                 I                                              -
  -                 I                                              -
 60-                I                                              -60
  -         *       I                                              -
  -                 I                                              -
  -                 I                                              -
  -                 I                                              -
 50- -----*--------* I ------------------------------------------ -50
  -                 I                                              -
  -                 I                                   *          -
  -                 I                                              -
  - *               I                                              -
 40-                I                                              -40
  -                 I                                              -
  -                 I                                              -
  -                 I                                              -
  -                 I                                              -
 30- --------------- I ------------------------------------------ -30
      ?   L   F   K I Hs   D   Hy  Pd   Mf  Pa   Pt  Sc   Ma  Si

Raw   1   4   6   12  13  34  25  25   30  13  29  21   13  44

K-Correction          6           5           12  12    2

T    41  50  58  49   70  92  65  76   69  65  87  71   45  71
```

Percent True :   42   F - K (Raw)   : -6
Profile Elevation :   71.4   Goldberg Index : 34

Welsh Code :   2*7"4801'5 36-9:   FL/K?:

172

The Minnesota Multiphasic Personality Inventory

SUPPLEMENTAL PROFILE

Client No. : 27   Report Date : 14-FEB-84   Page 4

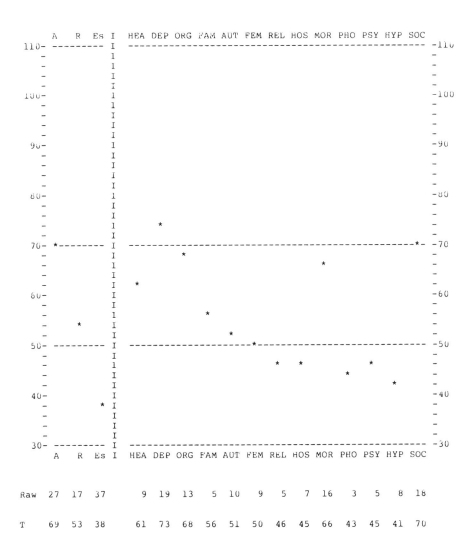

The Minnesota Multiphasic Personality Inventory

EXTENDED SCORE REPORT

Client No. : 27   Report Date : 14-FEB-84   Page 5

Supplementary Scales:	Raw Score	T Score
Dependency (Dy)	42	75
Dominance (Do)	13	45
Responsibility (Re)	20	50
Control (Cn)	26	53
College Maladjustment (Mt)	29	68
Overcontrolled Hostility (O-H)	9	38
Prejudice (Pr)	14	54
Manifest Anxiety (MAS)	30	71
MacAndrew Addiction (MAC)	22	50
Social Status (St)	20	55

Depression Subscales (Harris-Lingoes):

Subjective Depression (D1)	21	91
Psychomotor Retardation (D2)	9	70
Physical Malfunctioning (D3)	4	56
Mental Dullness (D4)	8	80
Brooding (D5)	7	76

Hysteria Subscales (Harris-Lingoes):

Denial of Social Anxiety (Hy1)	0	31
Need for Affection (Hy2)	5	50
Lassitude-Malaise (Hy3)	11	87
Somatic Complaints (Hy4)	5	59
Inhibition of Aggression (Hy5)	1	39

Psychopathic Deviate Subscales (Harris-Lingoes):

Familial Discord (Pd1)	2	51
Authority Problems (Pd2)	5	55
Social Imperturbability (Pd3)	4	35
Social Alienation (Pd4a)	7	56
Self Alienation (Pd4b)	9	70

Masculinity-Femininity Subscales (Serkownek):

Narcissism-Hypersensitivity (Mf1)	14	100
Stereotypic Feminine Interests (Mf2)	3	48
Denial of Stereo. Masculine Interests (Mf3)	3	51
Heterosexual Discomfort-Passivity (Mf4)	3	58
Introspective-Critical (Mf5)	4	55
Socially Retiring (Mf6)	5	49

Paranoia Subscales (Harris-Lingoes):

Persecutory Ideas (Pa1)	1	46
Poignancy (Pa2)	5	68
Naivete (Pa3)	3	46

Schizophrenia Subscales (Harris-Lingoes):

Social Alienation (Sc1a)	3	48
Emotional Alienation (Sc1b)	3	57
Lack of Ego Mastery, Cognitive (Sc2a)	5	72
Lack of Ego Mastery, Conative (Sc2b)	7	77
Lack of Ego Mastery, Def. Inhib. (Sc2c)	0	41
Bizarre Sensory Experiences (Sc3)	4	56

Hypomania Subscales (Harris-Lingoes):

Amorality (Ma1)	1	45
Psychomotor Acceleration (Ma2)	3	45
Imperturbability (Ma3)	1	36
Ego Inflation (Ma4)	3	52

Social Introversion Subscales (Serkownek):

Inferiority-Personal Discomfort (Si1)	22	110
Discomfort with Others (Si2)	3	43
Staid-Personal Rigidity (Si3)	7	39
Hypersensitivity (Si4)	7	80
Distrust (Si5)	9	77
Physical-Somatic Concerns (Si6)	5	79

The Minnesota Multiphasic Personality Inventory

CRITICAL ITEM LISTING

Client No. : 27   Report Date : 14-FEB-84   Page 7

   The following Critical Items have been found to have possible
significance in analyzing a client's problem situation. Although these
items may serve as a source of hypotheses for further investigation,
caution should be taken in interpreting individual items because they may
have been inadvertently checked. Critical item numbers refer to The
Group Form test booklet. Corresponding item numbers for Form R (only
items 367-566 differ) can be found in the MMPI "Manual" or Volume I of
"An MMPI Handbook." Corresponding item numbers for the Roche Testbook
can be found in "The Clinical Use of the Automated MMPI."

ACUTE ANXIETY STATE (Koss-Butcher Critical Items)

```
   3.  I wake up fresh and rested most mornings. (F)
   9.  I am about as able to work as I ever was. (F)
  43.  My sleep is fitful and disturbed. (T)
 152.  Most nights I go to sleep without thoughts or ideas bothering
       me. (F)
 186.  I frequently notice my hand shakes when I try to do
       something. (T)
 555.  I sometimes feel that I am about to go to pieces. (T)
```

DEPRESSED SUICIDAL IDEATION (Koss-Butcher Critical Items)

```
  41.  I have had periods of days, weeks, or months when I couldn't take care
       of things because I couldn't "get going". (T)
  76.  Most of the time I feel blue. (T)
  84.  These days I find it hard not to give up hope of amounting to
       something. (T)
 107.  I am happy most of the time. (F)
 142.  I certainly feel useless at times. (T)
 158.  I cry easily. (T)
 236.  I brood a great deal. (T)
 301.  Life is a strain for me much of the time. (T)
 318.  My daily life is full of things that keep me interested. (F)
 379.  I very seldom have spells of the blues. (F)
 418.  At times I think I am no good at all. (T)
 526.  The future seems hopeless to me. (T)
```

SITUATIONAL STRESS DUE TO ALCOHOLISM (Koss-Butcher Critical Items)

```
 137.  I believe that my home life is as pleasant as that of most
       people I know. (F)
```

MENTAL CONFUSION (Koss-Butcher Critical Items)

```
 328.  I find it hard to keep my mind on a task or job. (T)
 335.  I cannot keep my mind on one thing. (T)
```

356. I have more trouble concentrating than others seem to have. (T)

PERSECUTORY IDEAS (Koss-Butcher Critical Items)

278. I have often felt that strangers were looking at me critically. (T)

CHARACTEROLOGICAL ADJUSTMENT -- ANTISOCIAL ATTITUDE
(Lachar-Wrobel Critical Items)

28. When someone does me a wrong I feel I should pay him back if I can, just for the principle of the thing. (T)
38. During one period when I was a youngster, I engaged in petty thievery. (T)
250. I don't blame anyone for trying to grab everything he can get in this world. (T)
294. I have never been in trouble with the law. (F)

CHARACTEROLOGICAL ADJUSTMENT -- FAMILY CONFLICT
(Lachar-Wrobel Critical Items)

137. I believe that my home life is as pleasant as that of most people I know. (F)

SEXUAL CONCERN AND DEVIATION (Lachar-Wrobel Critical Items)

20. My sex life is satisfactory. (F)
37. I have never been in trouble because of my sex behavior. (F)
179. I am worried about sex matters. (T)
297. I wish I were not bothered by thoughts about sex. (T)
519. There is something wrong with my sex organs. (T)

SOMATIC SYMPTOMS (Lachar-Wrobel Critical Items)

36. I seldom worry about my health. (F)
55. I am almost never bothered by pains over the heart or in my chest. (F)
62. Parts of my body often have feelings like burning, tingling, crawling, or like "going to sleep." (T)
189. I feel weak all over much of the time. (T)
281. I do not often notice my ears ringing or buzzing. (F)
544. I feel tired a good deal of the time. (T)

NCS Interpretive Scoring Systems P.O. Box 1416, Mpls, MN 55440

MINNESOTA MULTIPHASIC PERSONALITY INVENTORY
Copyright THE UNIVERSITY OF MINNESOTA
1943, Renewed 1970. This Report 1982. All rights reserved.
Scored and Distributed Exclusively by NCS INTERPRETIVE SCORING SYSTEMS
Under License From The University of Minnesota

* "The Minnesota Report," "MMPI," and "Minnesota Multiphasic Personality Inventory" are trademarks owned by the University Press of the University of Minnesota.

Appendix E

Sample Report of Millon Behavior Health Inventory* with Computer Interpretive

The following report is generated after the patient responds to 150 true/false questions (not shown).

---

* Reprinted with permission of Interpretive Scoring Systems, a division of National Computer Systems, Inc.

MILLON BEHAVIORAL HEALTH INVENTORY
CONFIDENTIAL INFORMATION FOR PROFESSIONAL USE ONLY

REPORT FOR: SAMPLE C   SEX: FEMALE   AGE: 30

ID NUMBER: DATE: 16-SEP-83

CODE: - **8 * 2 6 1 5 + 7 4 3 "   //- **- * //NN**OO* //PPQQ**RR* //

```
****************************************************************
SCALES    * SCORE *            PROFILE OF BR SCORES          *
         *RAW  BR*     35    60    75    85          100 DIMENSIONS
*********+*******+--+-----+-----+-----+-----+------------+*********
        1  18   50 XXXXXXXX   |     |     |     |            INTROVERSIVE
        +--+-----+-----+-----+-----+-----+------------+
        2  13   70 XXXXXXXXXXXXXX   |     |     |            INHIBITED
        +--+-----+-----+-----+-----+-----+------------+
BASIC   3  15    9 XX         |     |     |     |            COOPERATIVE
        +--+-----+-----+-----+-----+-----+------------+
PERSNLTY 4 22   29 XXXXX      |     |     |     |            SOCIABLE
        +--+-----+-----+-----+-----+-----+------------+
STYLE   5  20   50 XXXXXXXX   |     |     |     |            CONFIDENT
        +--+-----+-----+-----+-----+-----+------------+
        6  15   63 XXXXXXXXXXXX     |     |     |            FORCEFUL
        +--+-----+-----+-----+-----+-----+------------+
        7  23   33 XXXXXX     |     |     |     |            RESPECTFUL
        +--+-----+-----+-----+-----+-----+------------+
        8  22   80 XXXXXXXXXXXXXXXXXXXXXXX   |     |         SENSITIVE
*********+*******+--+-----+-----+-----+-----+------------+*********
```

```
************************************************************************
* SCALES   * SCORE  *          PROFILE OF BR SCORES              *
*          *RAW  BR *    35    60    75    85   100  DIMENSIONS
************+***+***+-----+-----+-----+-----+-----+ 
         A   12   35  XXXXXX                          CHRONIC TENSION
         +---+---+---+-----+-----+-----+-----+-----+
PSYCHO-  B   14   70  XXXXXXXXXXXXXXXX                RECENT STRESS
         +---+---+---+-----+-----+-----+-----+-----+
GENIC    C   17   59  XXXXXXXXXXX                     PREMORB PESSIMISM
         +---+---+---+-----+-----+-----+-----+-----+
ATTI-    D   17   62  XXXXXXXXXXXXX                   FUTURE DESPAIR
         +---+---+---+-----+-----+-----+-----+-----+
TUDES    E   14   64  XXXXXXXXXXXXXX                  SOCIAL ALIENATION
         +---+---+---+-----+-----+-----+-----+-----+
         F   17   60  XXXXXXXXXXXX                    SOMATIC ANXIETY
************+***+***+-----+-----+-----+-----+-----+***************
PSYCHO-  MM  11   70  XXXXXXXXXXXXXXXX                ALLERGIC INCLIN
         +---+---+---+-----+-----+-----+-----+-----+
SOMATIC  NN  14   85  XXXXXXXXXXXXXXXXXXXXXXXXXXXX    GASTRO SUSCEPTBL
         +---+---+---+-----+-----+-----+-----+-----+
         OO  16   75  XXXXXXXXXXXXXXXXXXXXXX          CARDIO TENDENCY
************+***+***+-----+-----+-----+-----+-----+***************
PROG-    PP  20   97  XXXXXXXXXXXXXXXXXXXXXXXXXXXXXXXXXXX PAIN TREAT RESPON
         +---+---+---+-----+-----+-----+-----+-----+
NOSTIC   QQ  22   93  XXXXXXXXXXXXXXXXXXXXXXXXXXXXXXXX  LIFE-THREAT REACT
         +---+---+---+-----+-----+-----+-----+-----+
         RR   6   77  XXXXXXXXXXXXXXXXXXXXXX          EMOTIONALT VULNER
************+***+***+-----+-----+-----+-----+-----+***************
```

THIS REPORT ASSUMES THAT THE MBHI ANSWER FORM WAS COMPLETED BY A PERSON UNDERGOING PROFESSIONAL MEDICAL EVALUATION OR TREATMENT. IT SHOULD BE NOTED THAT MBHI DATA AND ANALYSES DO NOT PROVIDE PHYSICAL DIAGNOSES. RATHER, THE INSTRUMENT SUPPLEMENTS SUCH DIAGNOSES BY IDENTIFYING AND APPRAISING THE POTENTIAL ROLE OF PSYCHOGENIC AND PSYCHOSOMATIC FACTORS IN MEDICAL DISEASE. THE STATEMENTS PRINTED BELOW ARE DERIVED FROM CUMULATIVE RESEARCH DATA AND THEORY. AS SUCH, THEY MUST BE CONSIDERED AS SUGGESTIVE OR PROBABALISTIC INFERENCES, RATHER THAN DEFINITIVE JUDGMENTS, AND SHOULD BE EVALUATED IN THAT LIGHT BY CLINICIANS. THE SPECIFIC STATEMENTS CONTAINED IN THE REPORT ARE OF A PERSONAL NATURE AND ARE FOR CONFIDENTIAL PROFESSIONAL USE ONLY. THEY SHOULD BE HANDLED WITH GREAT DISCRETION AND NOT BE SHOWN TO PATIENTS OR THEIR RELATIVES.

COPING STYLE

THE FOLLOWING PARAGRAPHS PERTAIN TO THOSE LONGSTANDING TRAITS OF THE PATIENT THAT HAVE CHARACTERIZED MOST PERSONAL, SOCIAL AND WORK RELATIONSHIPS. IN ADDITION TO SUMMARIZING THESE MORE GENERAL FEATURES OF PSYCHOLOGICAL FUNCTIONING, THIS SECTION WILL BRIEFLY REVIEW THE MANNER IN WHICH THE PATIENT IS LIKELY TO RELATE TO HEALTH PERSONNEL, SERVICES AND REGIMENS.

BEHAVIORALLY, THIS PATIENT IS CHARACTERIZED BY VACILLATION, A PERSISTENT UNDERCURRENT OF TENSION ALTERNATING WITH OCCASIONAL PERIODS OF INTENSE MOODINESS AND ANXIETY, OFTEN EXHIBITED IN CRITICAL REMARKS. SHE FEELS BOTH MISUNDERSTOOD AND UNAPPRECIATED BY OTHERS, TENDING TO VIEW LIFE FROM A PESSIMISTIC AND DISILLUSIONED OUTLOOK. IN ADDITION, SHE IS HYPERALERT TO WHAT OTHERS THINK, AND ANTICIPATES THAT THE RESPONSES OF OTHERS WILL BE NEGATIVE. SHE EXPECTS THAT THINGS DO NOT GO WELL FOR VERY LONG. THERE IS AN INCLINATION TO REACT TO EVENTS IN A SOMEWHAT UNPREDICTABLE MANNER, WITH ANGER AND DISAPPOINTMENT EXPRESSED AT ONE TIME, FOLLOWED WITH GUILTY APOLOGIES FOR BEING SO EMOTIONAL THE NEXT. THIS EMOTIONALITY AND MOOD CHANGE IS BOTH PHYSICALLY AND PSYCHOLOGICALLY UPSETTING, AND MAY DISPOSE THE PATIENT TO AN INCREASED SUSCEPTIBILITY TO PSYCHOSOMATIC DISCOMFORTS AND AILMENTS.

PATIENTS SHOWING THIS PROFILE ON THE MBHI TEND TO VARY THEIR RESPONSE TO AILMENTS BOTH AS A FUNCTION OF THE NATURE OF THE AILMENT AND THE STAGE OR SEVERITY OF THE PROBLEM. AT TIMES THEY WILLINGLY REPORT SYMPTOMS IN AN ALMOST EXHIBITIONISTIC MANNER, COMPLAINING EXCESSIVELY ABOUT A VAST NUMBER OF DISCOMFORTS. THIS IS OFTEN EFFECTIVE IN GAINING THE ATTENTION OF DOCTORS AND OF FRIENDS AND RELATIVES WHO OTHERWISE REMAIN DISTANT. THESE PATIENTS TEND TO BE ERRATIC IN THEIR RELATIONS WITH DOCTORS, ALTERNATELY ENGAGING AND DISTANCING TO THE DISMAY AND ANNOYANCE OF THE HEALTH CARE PROFESSIONALS. THEY MAY COLLECT A VARIETY OF DOCTORS AND MEDICATIONS, SHOPPING ABOUT, RARELY SATISFIED WITH THE RESULTS OF ANY TREATMENT REGIMEN, OFTEN VOICING COMPLAINTS ABOUT THE QUALITY OF THEIR MEDICAL TREATMENT, AND COMBINING A VARIETY OF TREATMENTS AND MEDICATIONS WITHOUT SUPERVISION.

AT OTHER TIMES PATIENTS WITH THIS MBHI PROFILE WILL ACT IN A TOTALLY OPPOSITE MANNER, BEING FEARFUL AND ASHAMED OF THEIR SYMPTOMS AND INCLINED TO CONCEAL THEM. THIS RESPONSE MAY BE DISPLAYED BECAUSE THE SYMPTOMS OF THE ILLNESS RUN COUNTER TO THE SELF-IMAGE OF THE PATIENT. EXPECTING THE WORST, THESE PATIENTS ARE DISPOSED TO PROTECT THEMSELVES AND, THEREBY, BE HESITANT ABOUT EXPLORING THEIR AILMENTS AND RESISTANT TO EFFORTS TO HELP THEM. MORE IMPORTANT, BECAUSE OF THEIR FEARS AND PREOCCUPATIONS, THEY MAY BE TOO CONFUSED AND ANXIOUS TO UNDERSTAND OR FOLLOW MEDICAL ADVICE AND, THEREFORE, MAY NOT ADEQUATELY COMPLY WITH THE TREATMENT REGIMEN.

BOTH PATTERNS OF BEHAVIOR ARE EXPERIENCED BY A BUSY PHYSICIAN AS DEMANDING AND TIME-CONSUMING, OFTEN REQUIRING CONSIDERABLE PATIENT ATTENTION. HYPERSENSITIVE TO NEGATIVE SUGGESTIONS OR EXASPERATION, THE PATIENT WILL BE UPSET EASILY AND BECOME QUICKLY OFFENDED. EXPRESSIONS OF GENUINE SYMPATHY AND ATTENTION, HOWEVER, ESPECIALLY IF CONVEYED

WITH AN AIR OF CALM COMPETENCE, MAY HELP IN MODERATING AN UNJUSTIFIED OR HYPOCHONDRIACAL CONCERN ON HER PART. ALTHOUGH FIRM TIME LIMITS SHOULD BE SET TO CURTAIL EXCESSIVE DEMANDS, IT IS IMPORTANT TO MAKE SPECIAL EFFORTS TO COUNTER HER EXPECTANCY TO BE REJECTED AND TO FIND DOCTORS DISINTERESTED OR THOUGHTLESS. MEDICAL EXPLANATIONS SHOULD BE KEPT SIMPLE. THIS WILL AVOID AROUSING ANXIETY THEREBY COMPLICATING MEDICAL MANAGEMENT. REALISTIC AND ATTENTIVE REASSURANCES ARE A GOOD PRACTICE WITH THIS PATIENT.

PSYCHOGENIC ATTITUDES

THE SCALES COMPRISING THIS SECTION COMPARE THE FEELINGS AND PERCEPTIONS EXPRESSED BY THE PATIENT TO THOSE OF A CROSS SECTION OF BOTH HEALTHY AND ILL ADULTS OF THE SAME SEX. THE RESULTS OF THESE SCALES ARE SUMMARIZED HERE SINCE THEY MAY BE ASSOCIATED WITH AN INCREASE IN THE PROBABILITY OF PSYCHOSOMATIC PATHOGENESIS, OR WITH TENDENCIES TO AGGRAVATE THE COURSE OF AN ESTABLISHED DISEASE, OR WITH ATTITUDES THAT MAY IMPEDE THE EFFECTIVENESS OF MEDICAL OR SURGICAL TREATMENT.

THE PATIENT REPORTS LOW LEVELS OF PRESSURE RELATED TO THE DEMANDS OF FAMILY AND WORK RESPONSIBILITIES. THIS PERCEPTION OF AN EASY-GOING LIFE PATTERN SUGGESTS A LOW PROBABILITY OF TENSION-RELATED AILMENTS.

THE EVENTS OF THE PAST YEAR ARE REPORTED AS UNREMARKABLE AND TYPICAL IN CHARACTER FOR THE LIFESTYLE OF THIS PATIENT. PRONE TO VIEW EVENTS AS TROUBLESOME, THIS MODEST EVALUATION OF RECENT LIFE DIFFICULTIES SUGGESTS THE PATIENT HAS EXPERIENCED A MORE COMFORTABLE PERIOD THAN USUAL. THERE IS NO INDICATION, THEREFORE, THAT AN INCREASED PROBABILITY OF A MAJOR ILLNESS WILL OCCUR THIS COMING YEAR AS A CONSEQUENCE OF PERCEIVED LIFE STRESSES.

IN SPITE OF A CHARACTERISTICALLY PESSIMISTIC OUTLOOK ON LIFE, THE PATIENT RECOUNTS BOTH THE PAST AND THE PRESENT AS GOOD SOMETIMES, AND NOT GOOD AT OTHERS. THE INCLINATION TO INTERPRET EVENTS IN A REASONABLY BALANCED MANNER INDICATES THAT THE PATIENT IS LIKELY TO REACT TO AN ILLNESS EXPERIENCE IN AN UNEXCEPTIONAL MANNER.

ALTHOUGH USUALLY EXPECTING THE WORST, THE PATIENT SHOWS ONLY AN AVERAGE DEGREE OF CONCERN REGARDING FUTURE PROSPECTS. ASSUMING THAT THE OUTLOOK WILL UNFOLD IN AN UNEXCEPTIONAL MANNER, THE PATIENT IS LIKELY TO MANAGE FUTURE OR CURRENT PHYSICAL PROBLEMS WITH LESS EMOTIONAL UPHEAVAL THAN MIGHT OTHERWISE BE EXPECTED.

IN REPORTING ON THE CHARACTER OF FAMILY RELATIONSHIPS AND FRIENDSHIPS THAT MAY BE DRAWN UPON IN TIMES OF NEED, THE PATIENT DESCRIBES A LEVEL OF CONCERN THAT IS NEITHER EXCESSIVE NOR DEFICIENT. GIVEN THE CHARACTERISTICALLY NEGATIVE OUTLOOK OF THE PATIENT, THIS SANGUINE ATTITUDE IS A GOOD PROGNOSTIC SIGN AND SIGNIFIES THAT THE PATIENT ANTICIPATES ADEQUATE EMOTIONAL SUPPORT DURING PERIODS OF ILLNESS.

REGARDLESS OF OTHER DIFFICULTIES, THE PATIENT EXPRESSES NO UNTOWARD ANXIETIES REGARDING HEALTH AND ILLNESS. ALTHOUGH UNLIKELY TO OVERREACT TO ILLNESS ITSELF, THE MANAGEMENT ASPECTS OF A THERAPEUTIC PROGRAM ARE STILL LIKELY TO BE COLORED AND COMPLICATED BY THE CHARACTERISTICALLY NEGATIVE EXPECTATIONS OF THE PATIENT.

PSYCHOSOMATIC CORRELATES

The scales comprising this section are designed for use only with patients who have previously been diagnosed by physicians as suffering one of a number of specific disease entities or syndromes, e.g., hypertension, colitis, allergy. Note that these scales do not provide data confirming such medical diagnoses, nor do they include statements which may be construed as supporting them. Rather, the primary intent of this section is to gauge the extent to which the patient is similar to comparably diagnosed patients whose illness has been judged to be substantially psychosomatic, or whose course has been judged to be complicated by emotional or social factors.

Given a tendency to react strongly to feelings of tension, if the patient has a diagnosed allergic disorder, e.g., pruritis, urticaria, dermatitis, asthma, there is some basis for assuming that these reactions sustain or aggravate the disease process.

If the patient has a history of chronic gastrointestinal disorder, e.g., peptic ulcer, colitis, dyspepsia, irritable colon, there are strong indications that the characteristic emotionality of the patient, as well as possible new psychological stressors, have become major contributors to both the persistence and severity of the illness. Psychotherapeutic management is strongly recommended.

Consonant with the troubled view of life of the patient, if the patient has been medically diagnosed as manifesting the symptoms of certain cardiovascular disorders, notably hypertension or angina pectoris, it would appear that the physical discomforts felt by the patient are substantially influenced by stress.

PROGNOSTIC INDICES

The scales comprising this section have been empirically constructed to assist clinicians in appraising the impact of psychosocial factors which can complicate the usual prognostic course of patients who have a history of either a chronic or life-threatening illness, or who are under review for a life-sustaining surgical or medical procedure.

If there has been a medical history of a periodic or persistent pain disorder, e.g., low back pain, headache, TMJ, it is highly likely that the patient will not respond favorably to traditional outpatient treatment. Numerous complications are likely to arise during the course of treatment as a function of emotional responses to both the disorder and the treatment program. A conservative pharmacologic and surgical course is recommended. Serious consideration should be given to the option of behavioral modification programs and those utilizing other psychological treatment components.

If the patient is suffering from a chronic and progressive life-threatening illness, e.g., metastatic carcinoma, renal failure, congestive heart failure, MBHI scores would predict a substantially less favorable prognosis than average. The strong feelings of hopelessness, isolation and sadness make it imperative thatt psychotherapeutic or self-help efforts be undertaken to counter the destructive consequences of tthese forces.

If faced with major surgery or a candidate for ongoing life-dependent treatment programs, e.g., open heart procedures, hemodialysis, cancer chemotherapy, it is possible, although not probable, that the patient will suffer disorientation, a major depression or a psychotic episode. Counseling sessions both prior to and during treatment should minimize these possibilities.

CAPSULE SUMMARY

CONSTANTLY VACILLATING, MOODY AND CRITICAL, THE PATIENT OFTEN EXPECTS AND ELICITS NEGATIVE REACTIONS FROM OTHERS. FEELING POORLY TREATED BY HEALTH CARE PERSONNEL, SHE WILL EITHER OVERREPORT OR TOTALLY DENY SYMPTOMS. PROBLEMS ASSOCIATED WITH NONCOMPLIANCE AND THE UNWISE COMBINING OF MEDICATIONS SHOULD BE ATTENDED TO. REALISTIC, FIRM, YET CONCERNED ATTENTION, MAY MOTIVATE HER TO FOLLOW PRESCRIBED REGIMENS.

COPYRIGHT 1976, 1981 BY THEODORE MILLON. ALL RIGHTS RESERVED.

PUBLISHED BY INTERPRETIVE SCORING SYSTEMS,
A DIVISION OF NATIONAL COMPUTER SYSTEMS INC.
P.O. BOX 1294, MINNEAPOLIS, MN 55440

NAME: SAMPLE C   0050051

Index

A

Accounts payable programs, 17, 23
Accounts receivable programs, 25
Accounts receivable report (A/R report), 69
Aged receivables report, 113
Antistatic supplies and equipment, 43
A/R report (accounts receivable reports), 69
Arion, 126
ASCII, 36

B

Backup, 51, 55–58, 71–72
  floppy disk, 57
  hard disk, 57
  long-range, 57–58
BASIC, 28, 29
Bidirectional tractor, 98
Billing and collecting 1–2, 6, 124–126
Blank diskettes, 42
Blue Cross/Blue Shield, 10, 73–74
Bookkeeping, 21
Bytes, 31

C

Cables, 42–43
Cathode ray tube (CRT), 24, 40–41, 96
  office lighting, 82–83
Central processing unit (CPU), 28, 31–32, 95–96
CHAMPUS, 10, 73–74, 163–64
Charge transactions, 8
Check-writing, 23
Collections, 73–74, 124–26; see also Dunning system
Commands, 51
Communication hardware, 41
  cables, 42–43
Communication software, 17, 24
Compu-Psych, Inc., 126
CompuServe, 24, 131, 134
Computer, 95–96
Computer applications
  billing, 1
  scoring, 1, 3
  tracking accounts, 1, 3–4
  typewriting, 1, 2
Computer Readable Data Bases, 131
Computer reports on practice activity, 155–62

Computer service bureaus, 109, 111
Computer supplies, 53, 81–82
  list, 107–8
Computer system, 28–46
  communication hardware, 41
  CPU, 31–32
  keyboard, 28–31
  memory, 32
  money making potential, 117–27
  multi-user, 135–39
  myths, 59–64
  optimal use, 118
  physical considerations, 82–83
  preparing for use, 79–83
  printer, 37–40
  sequence of ordering, 81–82
  storage, 32–37
  use in office, 65–78
  video display, 40–41
Computer table, 45
CPU; see Central processing unit
CRT; see Cathode ray tube
Custom-made hardware, 87

D

Daisy Wheel printer, 37–40, 98
Data base management system (DBS), 17, 21, 49, 100, 121–23
  definition, 130
  Profile program, 95
  readable, 132–34
    efficiency, 133
    future, 133–34
    serious, 132
    time and charges, 132–33
  recreational, 132
  software, 20–21
Data racks, 46
Data trays, 46
Day sheet, 73, 109, 111, 155–58
Demographic reports, 12
Dental office system (DOS), 5–6
Diagnostic file, 7
Dictionary, 102
Disk drive, 15, 32–35
  storage boxes, 42
DMP 2100 printer, 98
Dot matrix printer, 37–40
Dow Jones Free Text Search, 130, 133

187

Dow Jones News Retrieval Service, 24, 29
Dunning system, 3–4, 100

E

Electrical requirements, 82
Electronic data base, 133
Electronic spread sheet, 24, 73
External computer system, 109–15
  advantages, 111–14
  disadvantages, 114–15
External data base (EDB), 24

F

Fanfold folders, 45–46
Financial recaps, 12
Financial reports, 10–12, 100
Financial spread sheet, 17
Floppy disk drive, 15, 33–34, 42, 97
  backups, 57
  labels and pens, 46
  maintenance and cleaning supplies, 43
Follow-up, 119–20
Furniture, 99
  configuration, 82

G–H

General ledger programs, 21
Grammar checking programs, 20–21
Green bar paper, 45–46, 69
Hard disk drive, 15, 33, 34, 97–98
  backups, 57
  speed, 63
Hardware, 41, 87
Health insurance claim form, 164

I–K

Information retrieval system, 130; see also Data base management system
Insurance forms, 2, 9, 10, 53, 70, 81, 164
Invoice forms, 82
Keyboard
  configuration, 28–29
  detachability, 30–31
  feel, 29
  Radio Shack Model 16, 96
Klein, Judy Graf, 38–39

L

Label printing, 15
Lighting, 82–83
Long-range backups, 57–58
Long-term storage, 32–33

M

Makover, Joel, 82 n
McWilliams, Peter, 30

Medical office system (MOS), 5–9, 17–18
  ancillary use of computer, 126–27
  billing and collection, 124–26
  charge transactions, 8
  diagnostic file, 7
  implementing, 15–16
  learning systems commands, 51
  money making potential, 117–27
  optimal use, 118
  patient file, 7
  payment transactions, 8–9
  practice file, 6
  procedure file, 8
  Radio Shack equipment, 99–100
  report formats, 9–12
    demographic, 12
    financial, 10
  software, 17–25
  sorting, 12–15
  starting up, 47–53
  stimulating patient/client interest, 118–23
  training, 49
  transaction file, 8
MEDLAR, 41
Memory, 32
Menu, 20, 66–67
Missed payment report, 112
MMPI scale, 3
Modem (Modulation-Demodulation unit), 41, 130
MOS; see Medical office system
Multiple disk drive, 34
Multi-user computer systems, 135–39

N–O

National Computer Systems (NCS), 126
Numeric pad, 29
The Office Book, 38–39
Open contract reports, 160

P

Patient file, 7, 67–68
Patient statements, 10–12
Payment transaction records, 8–9
Payroll systems, 17, 23–24
Power line protectors, 43–44
Practice file, 6
Practice management summary, 161
Previous accounts receivable, recording of, 50
Print commands, 20
Print ruler, 46
Printer, 37–40
  medical office, 39–40
Printer table, 45
Printer tractor, 44–45, 98

Index **189**

Procedure file, 8
Production analysis report, 162
Profile (data base program), 35, 95, 103
Program commands, 51
Programming, 80
Psychological office system (POS), 6
Psychological testing, 126–27
Psychometer, 126
PsychSystems, 126

R

Radiation, 41
Radio Shack, 92
  catalog, 93, 106
  computers, 95–96
  data base course, 95
  furniture, 99
  operator's course, 94
  printer, 98
  software, 99–103
  supplies, 103–8
  word processing course, 94
Radio Shack Direct Connect 1, 41
Random access memory (RAM), 32, 34–35
Readable data bases, 132–34
Recall, 118–19
Recreational data base, 132
Report format, 6, 9–10, 20–21, 23–24
Rorschach scale, 3

S

Safeguard Business Systems, Inc., 109–11
Scoring, 1, 3
Scripsit, 94, 102–3
Service contracts, 105
Slesin, L., 41n
Software, 17
  communications, 24
  data base management, 21–23
  general ledger, 21
  word processing, 18–20
Sorting, 12–15
The Source, 132
Spelling programs, 20–21, 102–3
Spread sheet, 24–25
Storage, 32–37
Submenu, 67
Supplies, *see* Computer supplies

T

Telenet, 130
Tracking accounts, 1, 3–4, 124–26
Tractor, 44–45, 98
Training, 49
  staff needs, 80–81
Transaction file, 8, 69
Turnkey operation, 4, 63–64, 85–108
  custom-made, 87–89
    costs, 88
    financial stability of supplier, 89
    hardware, 87
    proximity, 89
    support, 88
    time, 88
  do-it-yourself operation, 92–108
    equipment, 95–98
    furniture, 99
    instruction, 94–95
    service, 105–6
    software, 99–103
    supplies, 103–8
    support, 105
Typewriting, 1, 2

U–V

User-defined keys, 20
User modification, 99–100
Utility commands, 51
Video display, 37, 40–41, 66, 96
  radiation, 41
Visi-Calc, 24, 103

W–Z

Wechsler Scale, 3
Window, 20
Word processing system (WPS), 2, 18–20, 71
  grammar checking, 20–21
  menu, 20
  Scripsit program, 94
  spelling, 20–21
  training, 49
  window, 20
Zaks, Rodnay, 44
Zybko, M., 41n